Acclaim for Diana Raab's *Healing with words*

"*Healing With Words* offers unique therapy for cancer patients. Raab is a registered nurse, author, mother of three and a happily married woman. Her compelling and inspirational book reflects her two episodes with cancer over several years. She expertly tells her story and captures the reader with her feelings, frustrations and fears that overwhelmed her from the diagnosis of breast cancer through the reconstruction and recovery through her subsequent bout with multiple myeloma.

Descriptions of her personal journey are accompanied with powerful poetry and journal entries she wrote at various stages of her illness. What is unique about this book is that its messages are universal. Any cancer patient or survivor can relate to and learn from what she experienced.

Included in the masterfully written book are writing prompts to encourage readers to write about what is happening or has occurred in their lives.

As a college writing professor, I give Diana Raab an *A+* for her writing. As a two-time cancer survivor, Diana who has taught Writing for Wellness classes for patients at the City of Hope Cancer Center for eight years, I congratulate for her significant contribution to the field of writing-to-heal techniques. Her book is a must-read for any woman diagnosed with breast cancer."

Julie Davey, author,
Writing for Wellness: A Prescription for Healing

"Diana Raab has shared her breast cancer journey with such honesty that is truly compelling. Anyone receiving a cancer diagnosis should have *Healing With Words* to turn to time and again for comfort and guidance. Highly recommended!"

Beverlye Hyman Fead,
Legislative Ambassador and *Hero of Hope*
for American Cancer Society and author of *I Can Do This*

"*Healing With Words* is a riveting memoir which follows the author's journey through two cancer discoveries in eight years. Within the first thirty pages, tears filled my eyes as I felt Diana's pain and rebellion entering a new life, a new world. The book's structure allows the reader to find her own words to write beside Diana's enlightening story, which enlists it as a personal journal. Her poetic flavor of writing with lines like, 'My cancer diagnosis became like a stir-fry of emotions cooking inside me,' stretched my writer's mind and urged me to post my own note to my computer screen which was gleaned from this book, When it hurts—Write harder."

Barbara Sinor, Ph.D.,author,
An Inspirational Guide for the Recovering Soul and
Tales of Addiction: Stories from the Soul

"Although Diana Raab is a medical professional, she documents the recovery process also as a woman, daughter, friend, wife, and mother using words juxtaposed with journal questions, entries and poetry. One such poem, "A Woman's Life," uses 37 words to describe our many developmental stages. One of these is *writing*.

Writing is a gift that Diana shares with the reader. For any individual surviving a trauma, there need to be strategies and tools that can be utilized to help the individuals move from feeling like a victim to knowing that they are a survivor. Diana's book shares not only how writing impacted her journey, but also makes the suggestion that readers use writing as a process that can help to increase feelings of strength and personal power. This is a thoughtful book that will touch the hearts of women and those who love us."

Theresa Fraser, MA, author,
Billy Had to Move: A Foster Care Story

"Though I am a professional writer, it's hard to find adequate words for the admiration I feel for Diana Raab and her inspiring true story: *Healing With Words*. Time after time, Diana articulates incisively the thoughts and feelings that convey the hoped-for meaning and encouragement. She is a woman who knows what it is to live fully in the face of mortality. She will add value to the life of every person who reads this book. That she includes the creative impulse to write and the solace offered by contemplating the beautiful as a vital part of human existence resonates at a spiritual level for me."

Sena Jeter Naslund, author,
Ahab's Wife and *Abundance: A Novel of Marie Antoinette*

"One woman's story, beautifully told and inspiring to those for whom journaling will ease a breast cancer diagnosis."

Barbara Delinsky
New York Times bestselling author of *UPLIFT: Secrets from the Sisterhood of Breast Cancer Survivors*

Healing with Words

A writer's cancer journey

Diana M. Raab, MFA, RN

Loving Healing Press

Library of Congress Cataloging-in-Publication Data
Raab, Diana, 1954-
Healing with words: a writer's cancer journey / by Diana M. Raab.
p. cm.
Includes bibliographical references and index.
ISBN-13: 978-1-61599-010-8 (trade paper : alk. paper)
ISBN-10: 1-61599-010-0 (trade paper : alk. paper)
1. Raab, Diana, 1954- Health. 2. Breast--Cancer--Patients--Biography. 3. Bone marrow--Cancer--Patients--Biography. I. Title.
RC280.B8R323 2010
362.196'994490092--dc22
[B]
                              2009036523

Portions of this book previously appeared in:

"Conversation with Flowers," "Why I Love California," "Life Handed Me a Memoir," "Bifurcation," "Robbed Twice," "Java Genetics," and "Losing My Menopause," previously appeared in *The Guilt Gene* (Plain View Press, 2009).

"A Woman's Life," "Your Voice," "The Blues," "Message to My Family," "To Dettner," and "Dampened Creativity," previously appeared in *Dear Anaïs: My Life in Poems for You* (Plain View Press, 2008).

"After the Orchid Show," "To My Daughters," "His Piano," and "Naked," previously appeared in *My Muse Undresses Me* (Pudding House Publications, 2007).

Distributed by Ingram Book Group, Bertram's Books, New Leaf Distributing.

Published by
Loving Healing Press   www.LovingHealing.com
5145 Pontiac Trail   info@LovingHealing.com
Ann Arbor, MI 48105   Toll-free 888-761-6268

Dedicated to Simon

Contents

List of Poems

Disclaimer

The material in this book is intended to provide the personal medical journey of one woman with breast cancer. When the medical information was shared, every effort was made to provide accurate and dependable information. However, professionals in the field may have differing opinions in terms of treatments, and medical advances continue to happen. Any of the treatments, medical, homeopathic or emotional described herein should be undertaken only under the guidance of a licensed health-care provider. The author, editor, and publisher cannot be held responsible for any error, omission, professional disagreement, outdated material, or adverse outcomes that derive from the use of any of the treatments or resources shared in this book, either in a program of self-care or under the care of a licensed practitioner.

Acknowledgements

It is impossible to write a book like this without the professional and emotional support of important people in my life. It's also impossible to acknowledge all the names of those who crossed my path during these difficult years and inspired me to write this book. However, there are a handful of people whom I certainly could not have done without, in both my medical and literary realm.

These people include my medical and nursing support team whose encouragement and positive attitude helped me believe that I would survive and return to a vibrant and productive life: Mel J. Silverstein, M.D., Constance St. Albin, R.N., James Waisman, M.D., Randy Sherman, M.D., Soram Khalsa, M.D., Leonne Schillo, M.S.N., David Molthrop, M.D., Anne Claiborne, M.D., Clifford P. Clark, M.D. and Keith Stewart, M.D.

I thank my wonderful family for their unrelenting love through their presence, phone calls, flowers, chocolate, and inspiration, and their love that gave me the strength to beat this disease: Simon, Rachel, Regine, and Joshua, Alexandre and Jeannine Raab, Eva Marquise, Robert and Silva Marquisee, Jed and Karen Marquisee, David and Henia Nameri, Serena and Frank Goitanich, David and Kim Raab, Agi and Jack Mandel, Ivan and Genevieve Reitman, and in the loving memory of Lilly Berenhaut, Ernest Raab, Louis Marquisee and Barbara Provan.

Appreciation goes to my friends and writing colleagues who not only read the early drafts of this manuscript, but whose encouragement helped bring the project to fruition: Connie May Fowler, Richard Goodman, Cheryl Dellesega, Loren and Robert London and Joan Pohl. Also special thanks to Sena Jeter Naslund and Karen Mann for accepting me into the M.F.A. Program at Spalding University months after my diagnosis, and where ultimately this project was born. Thanks to my publisher Victor R. Volkman who believed in this project from the beginning, and who has been a pleasure to work with. And special thanks to Maggie Lang and Allison McCabe for their conscientious and caring editorial input and whose assistance in the final touches of this manuscript was invaluable. Special hugs to my dear friend Jean Harfenist for her insight and boundless love.

Last but not least, to all those people in this world who have, and continue to battle, the same demon.

Foreword

For the past forty years, my medical expertise has been exclusively in the field of breast surgery, and more specifically caring for women with invasive breast cancer and DCIS (*ductal carcinoma in situ*). DCIS is considered an early form of cancer where abnormal cells multiply to form a growth within the breast ducts but they have not yet invaded the surrounding support tissues. If left untreated, many DCIS will develop into invasive breast cancer requiring more serious treatments.

The author's cancer was detected early during a routine mammogram, generally the only way to identify this type of breast cancer. During her first visit to my Los Angeles office, I commended her on her diligence in tending to the results of her abnormal mammogram, because early detection and treatment are key to a good outcome.

In *Healing With Words*, the author shares her breast cancer journey in a wry, compassionate and professional way. She chronicles her story with poetic charm coupled with her nursing and teaching knowledge, a combination guaranteed to result in an engaging page-turner, while also offering tips, solace and encouragement for others who may find themselves in similar circumstances.

Throughout the book, the author stresses how writing has helped her cope, and she encourages readers to write. She also discusses the importance of orchids during her own healing and recovery. As her surgeon, I vividly remember her hospital room filled with their vibrant energy, which she claimed helped heal her spirit.

I applaud the author for having the courage to share her very personal story in the form of narrative, journal entries and poems. I understand that everyone reacts to and copes differently with the diagnosis of breast cancer and naturally everyone's story is unique, but this author's journey may serve as a guidepost for other women, motivating them to seek early detection.

The author describes, in simple terms, her medical and emotional journey, beginning with the news of an abnormal mammogram, to seeking out the best care, to six months later receiving her breast tattoo, and finally, to her very revealing afterword which further impresses the reader's appreciation of the author's commitment to this book.

Those who have dealt with cancer will say that the disease has transformed them, and this author is no different. However, what is remarkable is how she responded to her cancer after the initial shock wore off, and what's even more impressive is what she did with her transformation. The reader should observe and absorb and be inspired by her story, and how she did not let her cancer get in the way of her goals in life. On the contrary, her cancer gave her a reason to forge ahead toward her passions with determination and empowerment. Enjoy this profoundly supportive and inspiring story.

Melvin J. Silverstein, MD
Director, Breast Program
Hoag Memorial Hospital Presbyterian
Newport Beach, CA
Clinical Professor of Surgery
Keck School of Medicine
University of Southern California
Los Angeles, CA

Introduction

During my breast cancer journey, my lifeline was three-fold: immediate health care, an extremely supportive family, and the creative arts as a source of strength. For a long time, the arts have been associated with relieving tension and fears. Creative expression is a healthier alternative to keeping emotions bottled up inside or reaching for medications. Author Virginia Woolf confessed that she wrote in her diary "to bring order to the chaos in her life." Those of us who have been afflicted by cancer know there are no magic wands to take the cancer away, but we can try to cope with our situation and reduce stress by finding our passions, whether it is writing stories, crafting poems, journaling, drawing, painting or sculpting. If writing is your passion, then you understand how the very act of putting your words on the page is a productive way to ground you in your experience and give voice to your feelings. At times, you may find it difficult to express how you feel, but if you document your breast cancer journey, you will soon discover that your writing shines with power and beauty.

I have long understood the healing qualities of writing. Thus, it was no surprise that the first thing I did when returning home after my abnormal mammogram was to pull out my journal. From then on, I made a point to write early in the morning when my thoughts had the most clarity and purity. It is not essential to have a writing routine, but most writing instructors will advocate some sort of regularity, particularly in the beginning. In the writing classes I teach, I instruct my students that journaling is a reality check. Writing about the traumas in our lives is not only cathartic, but it can help provide answers to mysterious questions.

Journaling brings you face to face with your own truths and what has happened to you. The simple act of moving your pen across the page can be soothing and meditative. I used my journal to validate my feelings during my breast cancer journey.

For some people, it is difficult to begin the writing process, so for your convenience writing prompts are provided at the end of each chapter and in Appendix A. If you have borrowed this book from a library, I suggest you buy yourself a journal to write answers to the prompts. If you have bought this book, you can answer the questions right on the page, but you may also want to buy an additional journal for lengthier reflections.

I cannot over-emphasize the importance of journaling your feelings. After my surgery, my plastic surgeon encouraged me to write every day. He even asked me to mail him my musings. Because of their intimacy, there were certain things I preferred not to share. So in addition to the journal written especially for him, I kept one for myself, sections of which I have included in this book.

My journal also included poems crafted during and after my breast cancer journey. I have included most of them in this book, such as the poem below, inspired by a passion that began while I was in the hospital recovering from my breast surgery. All of the beautiful flower arrangements that filled my hospital room had died by the time I was ready to go home, all except for one white *phalaenopsis* orchid. In my heart, I took this as a message. I believed that like the orchid, I also would survive. I brought the plant home and placed it on my bedside table. As time went on, I became increasingly intrigued by its magic. Unlike any other flowering plant I had owned, it seemed as if it would bloom forever. In some parts of the world, orchids have been transformed into talismans, amulets, and good luck charms to ward off evil spirits, improve health, and help destiny take a more positive course.

I'd like to think they work, for it has already been eight years since I received the phone call informing me of my abnormal mammogram. In many ways it seems like yesterday, but in others it could have been a century ago. The journey of my diagnosis, treatment and recovery from breast cancer has been a life-altering event. When the fear gets overwhelming, my best remedy is to direct my creative energy to writing. I once had a writer friend who said, "When it hurts, write harder."

Those words remain on a Post-it® above my computer.

Conversation with Flowers

Slipping into my own dreams
I glance out the window
and spot the lavender
glistening under the energy of
another day going down,
touched by the evening vapors
ever so lightly in the night's breeze
waving another subtle good-bye.

When morning knocks,
I gently open the back door.
peak over the balcony's ledge
in anticipation of
the morning's dew once again
glistening on my lovely lavender.

I wonder if the bush ever sleeps,
or if it keeps busy watching
over me as I sleep.
The answer must be in its
everlasting fragrance
and in my dreams.

After the Orchid Show

Driving home two hours later,
sports car convertible down
crammed ten orchids high,
a warm welcome to this new obsession.
I stop at a red light, stare and sigh
at the lady slipper beside me. Its veined
pouch collects insects, the way I collect
your love in the arteries around my heart.

Its erotic glances paralyzing,
like the ones you toss over dinner
every Friday night to celebrate us.
You promise to plant an orchid
on my grave, the little green psychiatrist
which calmed me during difficult times
and which will bring me back again.

Truth is, I dreaded another plant
to care for or even let die. Water. Fertilize.
Water. Fertilize. But my new passion
pulled me in deeper, yanking me
to another focus, this marvel
of nature, mystified by rifles, thieves
and crazy characters.

1 Mammograms and More Mammograms

> "Those who don't know how to weep with their whole heart don't know how to laugh either."
>
> —Golda Meir

There is no breast cancer in my family. No cancer of any kind. Except for mine, that is.

Two days after my annual mammogram (I was a month late scheduling the appointment), the nurse phoned to say that the radiologist wanted to take additional views of my right breast. "He just wants to make sure that everything is okay."

This was not the first time I had been called back to the mammography department of my local hospital. A year earlier, I had had a surgical biopsy on the same breast, after a clinician detected a small lump during the manual examination before my mammogram. She had me sit on the edge of the examination table in my hospital gown during that fateful appointment, facing the mirror hanging on the wall. She asked me to raise my arms to see if she could detect any abnormal dimpling on my breasts. Then she asked me to lie down as she did the familiar circular examination that I did faithfully every month, on the first day of my menstrual cycle. I had cystic breasts, but the little cysts moved when I touched them. As a nurse, I knew that if a lump was fixed and did not move, then it was probably malignant and should be looked at right away. I never had any lumps like that.

"I feel a little lump here," she said gently, her hands still on my right breast. "Here, you feel it."

She took my index and middle fingers into her hands. "It's small and moveable, which usually means it's not cancer, but I'm sure they'll want to biopsy it."

Two weeks later I was admitted into the hospital for a biopsy. Thankfully it was benign.

So, when I received this second call from the nurse, part of me was pissed off at having to return for another false alarm. Although the biopsy was negative, the entire surgical ordeal was not something I wanted to endure again.

To be on the safe side, I booked the follow-up mammogram. The weeklong wait for round two was long enough for my imagination to go absolutely haywire. Studies were popping up in newspapers and magazines hypothesizing on what might predispose women to breast cancer. I tried to fit myself into a category, any category, that would indicate that I was at risk, but I could not. I had breast-fed all three of my kids, I exercised four times a week, ate lots of fruits and vegetables, avoided red meat, was not overweight, and drank lots of water. I visited a nutritionist regularly. I ingested a kaleidoscope of herbs and minerals three times daily. I was doing everything right. How could I have breast cancer?

On the morning of my appointment, the alarm rang at six a.m. I slammed the button, showered, and got dressed. My husband volunteered to accompany me to the hospital, but I said I would be okay going by myself. I kissed him good-bye and told him not to worry because it would probably be just another false alarm. What I did not say was that lurking inside of me was a growing sense that things would not be okay this time around.

I drove our twelve-year-old son, Josh, to school, then, hopped on the congested highway, heading to the women's health center. After parking in the hospital's early morning half-empty lot, I went directly to the radiology department, signed the receptionist's clipboard, took a number from the box, and sat in a waiting room crammed with women and old magazines splattered on laminated coffee tables.

Two out of the four magazines displayed headlines pertaining to breast cancer. My friend, Ellen, a radiologist, had (prior to my most recent mammography,) told me that the incidence of breast cancer had risen to epidemic proportions: one woman in eight would be diagnosed with it at some point in their life. This meant that whether at a dinner party or in a shopping center, chances are you would meet someone who already had breast cancer or would succumb to it later in her life. To me, this news was astounding. Another shock: 75 percent of new cases were not genetically related. It was this discussion that my mind kept casting back on. As I flipped through the magazines, pretending to read, my mind churned into a fast-paced movie laden with unanswered questions. *Do I have cancer? How will this affect our family?*

"Diana Raab," I heard the receptionist call my name.

A Woman's Life

Kicking
Wiggling
Sucking
Pushing
Nursing
Sleeping
Eating
Growing
Crawling
Sitting
Walking
Counting
Reading
Writing
Biking
Dancing
Flirting
Necking
Loving
Cramping
Rebelling
Driving
Exercising
Studying
Working
Marrying
Nurturing
Obsessing
Separating
Crying

Dieting
Menopausing
Wrinkling
Grouching
Forgetting
Slouching
Dying.

Describe your family and note if there is any history of breast cancer in your family tree.

Write about the day you first thought that you had cancer.

2 The Diagnosis

"Fear is an emotion indispensable for survival."
—Hannah Arendt

"Just move a tad bit to the left," the soft-spoken technician requested. .

Here I was again, wearing another paper gown (opened to the front) and back in the mammogram room having my boob squashed between two horizontal pieces of glass. I used my arm to hold onto the cold bar beside the machine, arching my back so the technician could get a good view of my (droopy) womanhood.

"Okay, hold your breath one more time," she said.

Then she dashed off to her protective cubicle. *Where is my protection?* I wondered. *Are they really certain all these mammograms aren't destroying my good cells?*

"Okay. Have a seat while I check to see if the films are good," she said, darting off to the darkroom.

I sat. I was hoping we were done, that my breasts would not have to endure any more torture. On the small coffee table beside my chair were pamphlets with graphic photos explaining how to give self-breast exams. *How many of those had I jammed in my purse during the past twenty years?* I wondered how many women actually took them out to read once they arrived home. Studies show that most breast cancers are detected by women themselves. Whatever was going on with me this time was definitely not palpable because my earlier scare made me diligent about performing the exams on the first day of each menstrual cycle.

After about fifteen minutes, the technician returned.

"Everything is fine," she said.

"You mean I am okay?" I said, with a certain degree of elation.

"No Ma'am, I cannot read your mammograms, I'm just saying the pictures came out." She hesitated. "The radiologist would like to talk to you."

"Is everything all right?" I asked.

"That's what he wants to speak with you about. Why don't you go get dressed and I'll meet you outside the changing room and bring you to him."

"Thank you." I quickly ripped off my hospital gown and slipped back into my black Capri pants and pink tank top. I embraced both my breasts and turned sideways in the mirror.

The technician was waiting outside the door.

I nervously followed her into a room lined with mammograms displayed on boards around a wall lit from behind. As I approached, the radiologist swiveled his chair around to glance up at me.

"Are you Diana?"

"Yes," I said with trepidation, walking toward him.

"Let's have a look at this together." He motioned me closer, and I felt my body get cold and my legs go numb. I tried stepping outside myself to become the clinical nurse I had been years earlier. If I didn't succeed, I would surely faint on the tile floor. I stood behind him as he pointed at the pictures of my right breast.

"I can't say for sure, but it seems to me you have something called DCIS, *ductal carcinoma in situ*."

He could have said anything and I still would have cried. My emotions were piqued. Before my biopsy the previous year, I was called back for repeat mammograms, but the radiologist never requested to meet with me privately. His decisions had been framed alone, behind closed hospital doors.

"This means," continued the radiologist, "there are some cancer cells in your ducts. My best suggestion is that you have a needle biopsy so that we can see the extent of the cancer."

My head felt light. The room began spinning about me. I asked for a chair and was given one by the nurse. The radiologist continued, "The only thing I really want you to know is if there's anything there at all, it's *extremely* early. You should have a degree of comfort in knowing that. The reason we wanted you to return for more films—and not wear deodorant—is that the first mammogram looked as if there was talcum powder sprinkled on your breast. We wanted to make sure that the spots were not from your deodorant."

I could not remember whether they had reminded me not to wear deodorant the last time.

"Now that you're not wearing any deodorant, we know that what we see are calcifications."

I thanked him. He handed me the mammogram envelope and suggested an appointment with a surgeon as soon as possible. I badly wanted to ask him to look at the films one more time so that he could rescind his diagnosis. Instead, the nurse returned to the room and asked if I was okay.

"Nope, would you be?" I blurted.

Perhaps she was sorry she asked. "Can I get you anything before you leave?" she replied.

"Thank you. I'll be okay." I answered.

I knew that I would not be okay.

I staggered out of the radiology department to the exit leading to my car. I sensed people's eyes upon me, curious about my demeanor. Once outside, I forgot where my car was parked. After walking a few circles, I found it. I opened the door and climbed into the driver's seat. I do not remember removing the keys from the lock or closing the car door. The sun shining in the front window provided no relief for my deep sense of bleakness. I plopped my head on the steering wheel and sobbed relentlessly. My eyes stung from the smudged mascara I had applied that morning. *For whom? The doctor?* After rubbing my eyes so hard that I could barely see out of them, I rummaged around in the back seat for used water bottles. I poured what little water I found onto a tissue to clean myself up, and phoned my husband at work. I sobbed copiously and my words slurred in his ears.

"I can't understand what you are saying—"

"I'm at the hospital. My mammogram wasn't good."

"What did it show?"

"Something called DCIS. It's an early cancer. Basically, it's a lot of calcifications on the breast. I want to see you," I said between sobs.

"Do you want me to come there?"

"No. I'll drive to your office."

"Are you okay to drive?"

"I'll be fine. See you in ten minutes."

I finished cleaning my make-up in the mirror, and then hit the road.

Simon closed his office door and led me by the hand to the leather sofa I had bought him years earlier for Valentine's Day. He took me into his arms and told me that he would do everything in his power to get me healthy. He squeezed me as tight as he did the day my father died twelve years earlier.

I never wanted to leave his arms.

My mother bestowed me with very few tidbits of useful information, but one was, "You should always have at least one doctor friend." So the following evening, I phoned Ellen, my friend the radiologist, who was also the director of mammography at our local hospital. Ellen and I had an extraordinary friendship that had taken seed several years earlier, during a fifth grade trip to Williamsburg with our daughters. We were blessed that our husbands also got along, so we often went out as a foursome.

"Diana, I'm so sorry you're going through all this. Do you have your films?" she asked with an equal amount of professionalism and empathy.

"I do."

"Then come on over right away," she said.

Ellen arrived at her front door, still in her business suit. She gave me a hug and invited me in. She took the mammogram envelope from my hand and with urgency in her stride walked to the dining room. One by one, she held each film up to a window lit by an outside garden light. I sensed she had performed this gesture many times before. She motioned for me to move closer.

"Let me show you something, Diana. This is your right breast. These lines are the mammary ducts. I think they're concerned about these white specks. They're calcifications."

I nodded.

"For the most part we all have some, and often that's okay. But, the problem is when they become more abundant. Do you have last year's films for me to compare?"

"I do," I said, removing them from the paper sheath.

"Okay, here we go," she said, holding the old films in her left hand and the new ones in her right as I held my breath, hoping she would say everything looked fine.

"Last year you had a few specks, but it looks as if there are more this year. That's why they're suggesting a needle biopsy."

She put the films down and wrapped her arm around my shoulders. "I want to send you to my friend, Phil, in Dallas; he'll take excellent care of you and will have your results right away." She glanced down at her watch, "It's too late now, but I'll phone him first thing in the morning. Promise. And then I'll call you. When's a good time for you to go to Texas?"

"A.S.A.P."

I was happy to have Ellen as a friend and felt fortunate to be able to take this trip. My husband's parents agreed to stay with our kids.

Who is the first person you told about your breast cancer? How did they react?

How are you feeling right now?

3   The Needle Biopsy

"You can't keep misery from coming,
but you don't have to give it a chair to sit on."

— Proverb

The following week Simon and I flew to Dallas. .We checked into the Dallas hospital's hotel room and the following day, my alarm clock shook us from bed at nine o'clock. It was the morning of my biopsy.

The waiting room for the women's health center was decorated with needlepoint chairs and rugs, nestled in a wood-paneled room. The receptionist sitting in this cherry-wood encased receiving area welcomed me, and handed me a clipboard with a stack of blank forms. I sat down beside half a dozen other anxious-looking women and their partners. My eyes shifted side-to-side, wondering what all those women were doing there. *Are they in a worse predicament than myself?*

Within moments a nurse called out my name. After flipping through my papers and making small talk about the weather, she directed me to the changing room—four barren cubicles containing clothes hooks and a small mirror. Outside these rooms was a cozy sitting area with magazines; the women waiting here were old enough to be my mother. *What am I doing here? Aren't I too young to have breast cancer?* I felt incredibly out of place.

When I left my cubicle, a middle-aged nurse came to direct me to the biopsy room. I desperately looked for a window into her thoughts. *Does she know what is going on inside me? What about my prognosis?* Her face offered no answers. Something about her smile did echo concern, but I did not know if her sentiments were directed toward me or toward all the women who stepped through the clinic's doors. *Maybe her face mirrors my fear?* As we entered the biopsy room palpitations chilled my chest. Tears fell upon my powdered cheek.

"Are you okay?" she inquired, closing the door and putting her arm on my shoulder.

"I'll be okay. I'm just nervous."

"That's normal. You're in good hands. Dr. Phil is the absolute best."

"Yes, I know. I came all the way from Orlando."

She nodded. "I need to take some chest measurements before we begin," she said, glancing at my breasts.

After untying the strings of the hospital gown, I looked down at my breasts too. The stretch marks were impossible to hide, a gentle reminder of having nursed three babies (coupled with sixty pounds of weight gain each time.) My areolas were fairly large and stretched out of shape. In one of the books piled on my bedside table, I had read (ironically, as it turns out) that breast-feeding is the best insurance against breast cancer.

My breasts had served me well. They were a sharp contrast to my 17-year-old daughter's perky ones, but they had nursed three beautiful children and brought me endless erotic pleasure. For me they were the perfect size for my five-foot-four small frame—tottering between and A and B cup-size. It never appealed to me to have them enlarged and I never made a fuss about them. They were there and once a month became a little more tender, but I never worried about that; it was expected, short-term, and part of being a woman. I sometimes wore camisoles instead of bras. *Maybe the lack of support contributed to their droopiness...*

"Okay, look straight ahead," the nurse said, while marking up my right breast with a pen.

There was a knock on the door and then it opened slightly. As Dr. Phil squeezed through the crack, I quickly closed my gown. He extended his arm, and a warm smile formed on his lips. He cupped both my hands into his. "What a pleasure it is to meet you," he said. "So you're good friends with Ellen?"

"Yes, and she recommended you very highly."

"How nice! We'll take good care of you here. So we're doing a needle biopsy on you today. Have you ever had one?"

"I haven't." A few years earlier when I had a cyst removed in the same breast, they did not do a biopsy first because it was so small and they were fairly certain it was benign.

"No problem. It goes fairly quickly, but the trick is you must remain completely still, and that's sometimes difficult for a long period of time. You don't have any back problems, do you?"

"None that I know of."

"Good, because you'll have to lie on your stomach for a little over an hour, and it could strain your lower back. Your breast will hang in an opening on the table and we will take the biopsies through that opening. "

He picked up on the uncertainty in my face.

"Don't worry, we'll anesthetize the part of your breast we're working on. But you might feel a little tingle now and then. Okay?"

He sat down in a swivel chair and faced my mammograms hanging on a lit screen.

"I suppose," I said. *What other choice do I have?* I reminded myself that he was one of the pioneers in performing this type of procedure.

"It looks as if you have some scattered calcifications," he said, turning back to me. "So we might have to take a few aspirations, just to make sure."

I parsed every word, listened to every intonation in his voice, and raked his face for any revealing expressions. Although he had a warm demeanor, in his eyes I sensed a reserved concern.

"Okay, let's start," he said. "I don't think you want to be in here any longer than you need to."

With my gown opened in the front, I stood on the stool beside the stretcher-like bed and gently put myself face down. I turned my head towards the wall. I really did not want to see what the doctor was doing. I tried lying as still as possible, and the long periods of silence were broken by Dr. Phil recounting each step of the procedure. Part of me wanted to hear all the details, yet another part of me did not. Some of his commentary froze me in the present and impeded my desire to daydream about more pleasant things in my life. Dr. Phil numbed my skin so I did not feel him taking any of the biopsies. I tried to repeat a mantra I had learned years ago during a meditation class.

Dr. Phil frequently asked if I was okay. I told him that I was fine. I think he was asking about my physical status and if I was comfortable. It was not the time to talk about how afraid I was to get the biopsy reports.

When he wasn't speaking to me I zoned out to recap my past and present and dream about my future. My life became a movie reel, and something inside me said that the film was running out.

"We're just about finished," he finally announced. "Why don't you get up into the chair so we can talk?"

As promised, the entire procedure had lasted about an hour. The nurse helped me up, and thankfully she cupped her arm under my armpit, as the room spun around me. She noticed the color leave my face and offered me orange juice.

As I sipped through a straw, Dr. Phil said, "I'm sure you want to know the findings. I cannot say they're good."

I motioned the cup down and the nurse took it from my shaking hand. I folded my cold and clammy hands on my lap. Because my husband was in the waiting room and not beside me paying attention, something he does so well, I had to carefully listen to Dr. Phil's words. The only way I could focus was to make believe he was talking about someone else— someone I did not really care about. The moment was too surreal for words.

"I took about twenty small biopsies. You have something called *ductal hyperplasia,* which means there are too many cells in your mammary ducts. This happens over the years and can be perfectly normal. But, sometimes the cells begin to look strange and we call this *intraductal hyperplasia with atypia.* If the cells keep multiplying in the duct and the number becomes very abundant, then it's called DCIS, or *ductal carcinoma in situ.* My suspicion is that's what you have."

"Now what?" I asked.

"At this point, I'd recommend a surgical biopsy which means that it would be done in the operating room and we would take a larger piece of breast tissue for analysis. Most often if the cells remain in the duct, DCIS may be reversed through hormonal treatments. The danger arises when the cancer cells break out of the ducts. When this occurs the diagnosis becomes invasive cancer, and surgery, possibly a mastectomy might be recommended. But, let's go one step at a time," he wisely concluded, seeing the horror sweep across my face.

After some silence, my eyes flooded with tears. My throat felt paralyzed. The questions did not roll off my tongue.

While seated on the edge of the examination table, Dr. Phil astutely put his arm around me. "For the surgical biopsy, I can recommend someone here. Or maybe you know someone in Orlando; it's your choice."

I tried taking a deep breath, but the air would not enter my lungs. *Did he clamp off part of my lung while he was doing the biopsy?* All I wanted to do was curl up on the examination table and remain there for the rest of the day. How could I face the world and the bombardment of phone calls from concerned friends and family members? I needed time to think, rehash, and protect my thoughts. The last time I had bad news of this magnitude was my miscarriage at the age of twenty-seven. My children's faces appeared before me. I had been on bed rest for each of the three pregnancies. My father's face popped out at me, and now ten years after his death, I was missing him more than ever. Tears fell when my grandmother's face appeared. I do not think I have ever been as close to another woman as I was to her. I thought about my husband and how I could never survive without him.

After gaining my composure, I pulled myself off the examination table. The nurse placed her arm around my waist, and repeated, "You are truly in good hands." She gave me a pitying and empathetic smile. Dr. Phil shook my hand and said, "I'm sorry."

As if I had already lost a breast.

Or had begun preparing for my own funeral.

I sensed he had already ascertained my prognosis, but he did not want to be the one to spill the news. I stared at him as if this would get him to talk, tell me more about what was going on inside of me. Instead, he wished me well and a safe trip back to Orlando. In slow motion, I walked toward the changing room, holding the strings on my flimsy hospital gown. I slammed the cubicle door shut and glanced at my curves in the mirror. It was my body, my very own that I had

had for forty-seven years. Just above my pubic-line was a ten-inch scar, shaped like a smiling face, the aftermath of three cesareans and three beautiful children. My right breast had a still-healing red scar from the needle biopsy that had doubled in thickness since its inception the year before. Friends and strangers proclaimed that I looked young for my age. None of this really mattered now. All of those compliments were diminished in the face of the news I'd just received and by what would be my agenda for the next few months. I could not bear the thought of being hacked up by surgeons again. I craved the silky scar-free body of my adolescent years.

The nurse walked me back to the waiting room, where my husband sat on the leather sofa reading *Newsweek.* He sensed my presence and looked up. I did not have to utter a word. He stood up, hugged me and said, "Shit, it's not good."

"No, it's not." My throat closed up again.

"Don't worry," he said, "the doctor came out to speak to me. You don't have to repeat everything. He was very thorough. We are going to get this taken care of. I promise—even if it means traveling to the other side of the world. We'll get it done."

My eyes swelled with tears. His words soothed me and I felt so blessed to have him, not only then, but always. *What would I do without him?* I thought of being there at that moment, all alone, with no one to hug or console me—like some of the other women in the room, awaiting their turn to see the doctor.

"The good news, honey, is that you're getting it looked after," said Simon. "Plus there's nothing you could have done different. Dr. Phil said that you could not have found this type of cancer on your own. It could only have been detected on a mammogram. We are doing everything we can do and moving as quickly as possible."

I would not want to survive without Simon. I knew this the moment our eyes met on his parents' balcony twenty-nine years earlier. My tears became a blend of happy and sad.

"Please don't blame yourself. Let's get you something to eat. You look pale."

"I'm not hungry, but you must be. I'll keep you company," I said in between waves of sniffles.

We found the hospital coffee shop and sat side by side in a booth. Simon did not stop caressing me. The intensity of his hugs pierced my core and massaged my pain.

While walking back to our hotel room I used my cell phone to call Ellen with my results. She asked if I wanted the surgical biopsy done in Orlando and I said no because I really trusted the expertise of doctors elsewhere.

"I know someone good in Dallas, if you like. But, why don't you come home and you can think about it in the meantime?"

The day after arriving home, I began my research. There was no one in my family to phone for a recommendation. The Internet was packed with information—lots of cold hard facts, but that was not what I wanted, nor what I was ready for. I was hungry for information from other women, women who had been through a similar scenario. I needed warm, compassionate, and real information. I phoned a childhood friend living in California who had been diagnosed with breast cancer the year before.

"Do not go for a surgical consult," she said, "because surgeons always want to operate. You need to find yourself a good oncologist. He'll tell you the absolute truth." What she was saying made a lot of sense. Even though I was a nurse, I did not think of this before she told me.

I phoned one of my favorite physicians in town—a urologist whom I had known for ten years. I knew that his wife had recently died of breast cancer. Certainly that experience, coupled with his genuine empathetic personality, would elicit the best assistance. He willingly recommended his wife's oncologist in Orlando.

A few days later I entered this oncologist's oblong waiting room. After signing my name on the clipboard on the ledge of the sliding glass reception area, I found a seat. All around me (again!) were mostly seniors, nursing their walkers or canes. They looked at me as if they were wondering what such a young person was doing there. I wondered the same. After flipping through the large-print *Reader's Digest* for a few minutes, I heard the nurse call my name.

Once in the examination room I had a pleasant surprise. The oncologist was a good-looking, tall man in his mid-forties. He seemed calm and positive. And he reminded me of one of my favorite TV doctors, Dr. Kildare. As a kid growing up in the sixties, I had a crush on him (and Dr. Casey.)

He held my mammograms up to the lit wall unit and invited me to sit on the examination table. Then he looked me in the eyes. Something about him was so connected, so much in my shoes. He made me feel as if I was his most important patient. After shaking my hand and introducing himself, he wisely said, "So tell me what they have already told you."

"They said I have DCIS and they recommend a surgical biopsy. I am here for your opinion."

"Looking at your films, I can definitely say that's what you have. I do agree with what you've been told. We will not know the extent until a surgical biopsy is done."

With my legs still dangling off the examination table, my feet felt a rush of cold. I had hoped that he would veto the possibility of anything being wrong with me. Oncologists were supposed to be more conservative than surgeons—that's what my friend had said. But he was sending me for a biopsy, too. Suddenly the small examination room began closing in around me. I turned to glance out the window through the slatted horizontal blinds. I wanted to jump out. He split the silence with a question.

"Tell me," he continued. "Do you travel at all?"

"Yes," I whispered. "I love traveling. I do a fair amount."

"Well, if it's not an issue for you, I would highly recommend you take a trip out to see Dr. Silverstein. He practices at USC in Los Angeles. It's far away, but he's tops in the field." He hesitated, and glanced back at my mammogram. "If you pick up any book on DCIS, his name is in it. He has done an enormous amount of research, and he lectures around the world. He's very well respected in surgical arenas. There are only a handful of breast surgeons. He's the absolute best."

"Traveling would be no problem," I said, numb.

He gave me the necessary phone number and confessed that if I were his wife he would recommend the same. I felt like hugging him.

When Simon and I returned to our hotel I immediately phoned the airlines for the earliest direct flight out to Los Angeles. Simon asked to accompany me, but I told him I would be okay. "It's just a consult appointment. If he suggests surgery I want him do it, and then I would want you to be there too," I said.

Your Voice

The sound of your voice
is like honey in my morning coffee

sunlight extending across the Pacific,
a vestal snowfall on a crisp Saturday,

the peeking through of the first spring flower,
smell of a newborn baby, of an acceptance letter,

love sounds in the night, the wagging of my puppy's
tail, piping hot maple syrup on pancakes,

cracking open your newly released book,
the look of a rushing waterfall, the regal

mountains, the snapping of an open fire,
gooey marshmallows on fraying sticks,

the warmth of your arms which promised
to hold me all century long, until we see

the next turn of the zodiac when we learn
we were born and will die under the same star.

What was the first thing that you thought of when you were
told that you had breast cancer?

How did you find your oncologist and/or surgeon? Who referred you? Describe your first meeting.

Was your oncologist optimistic about your prognosis?

What was your relationship like with your oncologist? Did you feel it was easy to talk to him or her? Were they accessible?

4 The Surgical Biopsy

"I feel like we are all islands—in a common sea."
—Anne Morrow Lindbergh

I was able to get an appointment with Dr. Silverstein for the following week. .From my hotel near the hospital, I hopped into a taxi, which dropped me at the doorstep of The USC Norris Cancer Hospital where Dr. Silverstein served as the Director of the Lee Breast Center.

I approached the rather small entrance to this grand institution and a security guard pulled open the double-glass doors. A bald woman in her forties, *like me,* was being pushed out in a wheelchair. Her left forearm housed an intravenous drip. She smiled a knowing smile in my direction, as if she remembered her first appointment in this building. My face must have been shadowed in fright.

I loved my breasts and was proud how they had nursed all three of my beautiful children. I loved my hair and never wanted to glance in the mirror to see that it had fallen out. I refused to accept that abnormal cells were proliferating inside me, wanting to control me, wanting to run my life. While studying in nursing school twenty-five years earlier, I learned that cancer patients were introverted and unhappy. *Was I like that?*

Once inside the main entrance, I glanced left and right and walked toward the reception desk. After I signed in, a friendly young man behind the counter pointed me across the hall to The Breast Center. The light and airy atmosphere soothed my fragile nerves. The place appeared clean, calm, bright and friendly. The staff wore white lab coats and smiled as they walked by. *Are they always like that, or do they see the terror in my face?*

I passed a gift shop with rows of small stuffed animals pressed against the window. From a string above hung socks, shirts, scarves, hats, and wigs of every style and color. A little further along was a clothing shop for post-mastectomy patients, featuring specialty bras and fancy hats. I walked quickly past these shops, glancing at them only through the corner of my eye, as if looking directly would bestow me with a fatal contagion.

I made my way to the waiting area. To me it was a good sign that I was the only patient. I sensed that is was a well-organized office. Within five minutes, Dr. Silverstein's nurse came to greet me. She was a bubbly woman about my age, and I could see trendy clothes peeking through her lab coat. She emanated compassion and warmth. Something about her made me feel comfortable. I remember thinking that she was the type of friend I would like to have. Our eyes linked, and I felt as if I had known her for years. "Hello Diana, I'm Connie, Dr. Silverstein's nurse. It's so nice to finally meet you. How was your flight?"

"No problem, thanks," I said, flattered that she knew who I was.

"You look good. You look like you live in Florida, tan and all."

"Thanks," I replied.

"I have some paperwork for you, and the doctor is ready to see you whenever you're ready." Out of the corner of my eye I spotted a tall gray-haired gentleman wearing large teardrop eyeglasses. His shoulders were somewhat slumped, perhaps the result of performing many surgeries. On his way to the computer set in the hallway, he waved and said, "You must be Diana."

"Yes, I am," I replied, surprised that he also knew my name. My mother always told me that you do not have the chance to make two first impressions and my first ones about the staff here were extremely positive.

I was escorted to an over-sized examination room with a rolling blackboard at one end. The large window overlooked the parking lot. I took it as another good sign that there were no magazines in either the waiting room or the examination room. There was no waiting time and therefore no time to read. For a split second, Connie walked out and then re-entered and stayed with the doctor during my examination.

"Hello, I'm Dr. Silverstein," he said as he came into the room, extending his rather long arm, offering me a strong handshake. He was the unassuming man I had seen moments earlier. His shake was solid—something my father always told me was a good thing.

"That means the person has character and is a trusting person," he told me. "Beware of fish-like handshakes. You want to watch out for those people." (What he did not tell me was that in certain cultures women often get gentler hand-shakes, so over the years I have learned not to generalize about such things, but I do keep all his words of wisdom in my thoughts.)

"So, what brings you all the way out to LA?" he asked, smiling.

I hesitated. "A consult with you!"

His smile widened and his glasses slid down his nose. There was something gentle about this surgeon; he did not seem the type of guy who would toot his own horn, nor did he seem to beat around the bush. If you met him anywhere other than his office you would likely not suspect that he was one of the world's most renowned breast surgeons.

"All the way to L.A. How lucky I am!"

I nodded. I liked his non-nonsense, warm personality.

"So I hear you have DCIS. You know that's my specialty?"

"I do. I'm here because I want your honest opinion. I know you're a surgeon, but if possible I'd like to avoid surgery."

"I can't blame you. How do you know you have DCIS?"

"It was detected through a needle biopsy."

"I see," he said, holding up my mammograms. "I suspect these have been looked at a few times," he said, pointing to a slew of fingerprints on its edges.

You got that right. "Yes."

While still focusing on the films, he asked how I heard about him.

"My oncologist in Orlando who's heard you speak at various conferences."

"He told you to come all the way out here? I'm sure there are good surgeons in Florida," he remarked, humbly.

"He spoke very highly of you."

"You do have DCIS, and from what I see, it's fairly widespread, although I've seen a lot worse."

My jaw muscles went slack. None of the other doctors mentioned anything about it being *widespread*. "And that means?" I asked.

"It can mean a number of things, but I can't say anything just yet. I suggest a surgical biopsy. Did they explain DCIS to you in a way you understand?" he asked.

"Yes, but I'd rather hear it from you."

"I suppose you've done some reading. All nurses do. But let's review anyway."

I suspected that Connie had told him I was a nurse, because I made no mention of it to him. I must have told her when I was making the appointment. There's a certain professional courtesy that comes with the territory of being in the medical profession, so when necessary I mention it.

He sat down and then slid his chair toward the blackboard on the other side of the room.

"Okay, let's say these are your breasts." He drew two droopy figures. I am not sure I appreciated being depicted in this way, but I suppose that wasn't the point.

"Your breasts have mammary ducts running through them," he said, drawing squiggly lines. "What you have are atypical cells growing in those ducts. These atypical cells are considered a type of pre-cancerous condition. My concern is that these cells have broken through the walls of the ducts. If this is the case then your cancer would be considered invasive and that's not a good scenario."

I felt the color leave my face.

Constance headed to the sink for a cold cloth. She signaled for Dr. Silverstein to slow down.

It was particularly painful hearing another person speak about something wrong with my breast. For some reason hearing bad news from Dr. Silverstein made it seem more real. "There's no need to worry yet," he said reassuringly. "I'll only know all the answers after doing the biopsy. For how long are you in town?" he asked.

"Until Thursday."

"So we have two days. I'd like to get you in while you're here so you don't have to do the back and forth thing." He turned to the nurse. "Connie, can you check my OR schedule?"

Within moments, Connie returned, holding his schedule, saying that he could do the biopsy early Thursday morning. A part of me wanted to get it over with, yet another part needed Simon beside me. My mind raced through the decision-making process. My breast was such an identifying mark of my womanhood. I wished we were discussing cutting into my gallbladder or small intestines, or something like that. I told him I wanted to speak with my husband. I truly felt incapable of making the decision without his input.

I walked outside and phoned Simon. He encouraged me to stay and have the biopsy. Luckily, my daughter Regine, who was fifteen, was in Los Angeles finishing up an art program at Otis College. We arranged for me to take a taxi to the hospital for the early morning biopsy, and she would meet me afterward and bring me back to the hotel. We would stay in Los Angeles for two days together.

The procedure went quite well, particularly since they put me under general anesthesia. It was quite similar to the surgical biopsy I had years ago with my false alarm on the same breast. Dr. Silverstein told me he would have my results only after I returned to Orlando, because the tissue had to be sent to a special laboratory. So Regine and I boarded the red-eye back home to Orlando. It was Saturday, August 11th, 2001.

Why I Love California

Dedicated to M.S.

Five years ago
I found myself
under the knife
of a fine surgeon
only days after
my diagnosis
of what strikes
one in eight women
arriving in this western
community to save me
from what could have been.

Did you decide to go for a second opinion and if yes, what did they say?

How did you feel after receiving a second opinion and how did it affect your decision/s?

5 The Results

"Life isn't a matter of milestones but of moments."
—Rose Fitzgerald Kennedy

On Sunday evening, August 12th, the phone rang. .
"Hello, this is Mel Silverstein." Intuitively I sensed that he was phoning with bad news; there was a tone change from when we met in Los Angeles. *Was I anticipating the worst? Was my pessimism surfacing?* I felt like ducking under my office desk as we used to do in elementary school to protect ourselves from nuclear warfare. I wondered if anyone ever hid under a desk to protect themselves from cancer.

I wanted to hang up the phone and let someone else do the listening, yet a corner of my psyche whispered that I should hear what he had to say. I took a deep breath.

"Well, Diana, there's good news and bad news. Is your husband with you?"

"Yes." I lost all my sense of focus and concentration. "We are both here. We'll put you on speakerphone."

"Hello Simon, this is Dr. Silverstein. I'm calling to give you both the biopsy results that just came in. As I was telling Diana, there's good news and bad news. The biopsy did show DCIS—quite diffuse around the breast."

Although I was beside the phone, I felt myself slip out of the moment, far away into some other land. Dr. Silverstein's voice became the background sound to my consciousness. It was as if I had stepped outside of myself. He could have been speaking about someone else, not me.

"As I explained to Diana," he continued, "DCIS or *ductal carcinoma in situ* means that small cancer cells have begun to settle and grow in your mammary ducts. As far as I know there is only some slight micro-invasion, but how extensive the micro-invasion is, I really won't know until more surgery is done."

As soon as he uttered the words, "more surgery," I was lost. Denial overpowered me, and all my life's fears began whistling true. This type of surgery that would remove one of my breasts was my worst nightmare. Being a nurse made me even more petrified. I knew and understood all that could go wrong with this kind of procedure. Plus, weren't one miscarriage, three cesareans and a knee surgery enough? How could one person endure more than that? *And why me?*

Would there ever be peace in my life? I wanted to curl up and call it quits.

Dr. Silverstein's and Simon's voices became a blur of dialogue echoing through my speakerphone. My mind denied everything they said about my forty-seven-year-old body. For a split second I wondered if Dr. Silverstein mixed his patients up and perhaps had phoned me instead of some other poor soul. I desperately wanted that to be the case.

I gazed out the window as if the swaying bamboo could cast some clues as to what this was all about. I looked beyond to the blue sky sprinkled with clouds as the sun began setting upon the horizon. I had never prayed, but I looked up into the heavens and pleaded with my father to make sure everything would go all right.

My eyes turned back toward the phone, and then to my husband's eyes, and then to the black and white school photos of our three kids hanging on the wall and the innocence and love in their eyes. I could not focus on Dr.

Silverstein's words. All I kept thinking was, *"This must be a mistake."*

I allowed Simon's ears and voice to take over. After half an hour of hearing, but not really listening, I managed to scribble a few words onto my yellow pad, about DCIS and needing to have surgery. We thanked Dr. Silverstein, disconnected the call, and simultaneously plunked onto the office sofa.

Simon drew me close, holding me tight. I wallowed in his strong arms. For about five minutes, silence reverberated in the room, until he blurted out, "fuck." We looked at one another and collided foreheads as if the motion would make the news sink in or simply make it go away.

I wanted to be dead. That must be a better alternative to mutilating the part of me that nursed and nurtured all three of our children, the part of a woman symbolizing womanhood, the part men glance at when not noticing my eyes first. I had an overwhelming sense of helplessness. I would never take my life, but for the first time I got a glimpse of what it might be like to be on the cusp of that action.

My memory rushed back to the day Rachel was born, and how I had prepared my breasts for her arrival—rubbing the nipples each night with a washcloth to get them callused. I meditated on my excitement to breastfeed her, to do something my mother found revolting, something she equated with primitive cultures or those more economically challenged. I thought about how my dreams of breastfeeding became shattered when Rachel was born prematurely, and upon the endless hours using the breast pump in the hospital, and filling bottle after bottle to feed her, offering the best a mother could offer. I thought about the ease with which my next two children nursed. I thought about their excitement— the kicking and wiggling at the mere scent of me, eagerly waiting for the placement of my nipple into their little mouths. I thought about how articles in women's magazines and books on my nightstand promised that breastfeeding would decrease my chances of ever developing breast cancer. *Bullshit!*

Images of masked surgeons glancing down at my bare, middle-aged body haunted me. Which medical residents would learn at my expense? I had done my fair share of nursing internships in operating rooms. I imagined myself on the other side of the chaos, lying on the operating room table listening to the laughter, the successes and the goof-ups. Nausea crept up into my throat.

Simon told me he loved me and would always love me. I never doubted his love, but still wondered how I could be blessed with such a terrific man, and how he could put up with the shit I had put him through—three pregnancies laden with bed rest and caesareans, colicky babies, migraine headaches, knee surgery, and now breast cancer. He said that was what love was all about, and he knew that I would do the same for him.

For the first five years of our love affair Simon had struggled to get me to express myself verbally. It was impossible for me to say what was on my mind. He had to yank my thoughts and feelings out of me. It was not easy; I had been raised in a home where the chance to speak my heart was not encouraged, and if I attempted to do so, I was quickly quieted. We are products of our childhoods; being mocked for my insights became my largest fear in life. Perhaps that is why I became a writer. For years, my only means of communication was on the page. Half my childhood was spent sitting in my walk-in closet writing in my journal. That was my way of sharing the emotional truths nestled in my soul. It was impossible for me to cross any boundaries with the spoken world. But, after thirty years together and a great deal of love and patience, Simon has taught me to speak my mind. (I am sure there are times when he is sorry he succeeded!)

Now, still seated on the sofa, Simon caressed both my breasts. He vetted them carefully and then said what he used to tell me earlier in our marriage. "More than a handful is a waste," hoping to get a chuckle.

At that moment, I craved having more than a waste. I felt every throb, every tingle, and every squeeze. I wanted to flood my memory with those sensations. Instead of levity, I spoke my mind and asked him to repeat Dr. Silverstein's conversation. Two of his words continued echoing in my head—"cancer" and "mastectomy."

Filling in the blanks petrified me.

All three of my children were home, and seeing them pass in the hallway saturated my eyes with tears. *How could they live without me?* My life had been determined by them... and theirs by me. Simon and I fell in love as teenagers and our love has blossomed beyond bounds. *How could we all live without one another?*

Simon stood up and closed our joint-study door. "Honey, this is a shock. I was not anticipating that phone call. Ever. He said you had DCIS and it is fairly widespread. If he was to excise most of it, it would leave your breast severely deformed, and afterward you would need chemotherapy and radiation. So he's suggesting a mastectomy and reconstruction instead."

Tears filled my eyes. *A mastectomy.*

Simon pulled me in closer. "That's what Dr. Silverstein would do if you were his wife. He also mentioned a plastic surgeon who works closely with him. He said you should give him a call."

Simon knew that it was impossible for me to absorb any more information than that. He would save the rest of the details for later. In my heart, I pinned my hopes on the chance that not discussing them would perhaps make the issues disappear.

"Why me?" I asked. It was a creepy feeling knowing cancer was growing inside me, that it had been lurking there. "There's no cancer in my family!"

"I don't have the answer to that. I don't understand either."

Shivers overtook my body but did not fend off the awful thoughts. My mother used to work as a receptionist in the office of an internist who believed that cancer patients keep their emotions and anger locked up inside them. His theory did not make one bit of sense to me back then, and I had always denied the negative stigmas associated with cancer. Yet at that moment, I wanted to grasp onto any theory that would promote my understanding of this illness.

Laws of Attraction

In seventh grade
my physics teacher
took us on his sailboat.
He was a tall blue-eyed,
gray-haired guy
with a smile which
could power his vessel.

Dr. Cotton's lightness of being
pulled me in like the inertia
he professed. It's no wonder
that twenty years later I fell
for another physicist who
taught me that life
is all about energy.

The Blues

You may think
I like the music
or the rhythm of the band,
but of what I speak
is the sadness which engulfs
my spirit in this gloomy isolation
of unexplainable origins.

A dizzying sense of blackness
churns about me. I see
no wonders created here.
My tears swell like the foam
of the cappuccino which opens
my eyelids each morning
when I really don't want
to face another day of loneliness.

I hunt for a place to turn, but am blinded
by doors slamming around my ventricles
and as my heart is squeezed like a girdle
to useless hips. I am blinded
by my pain and realize that it's time
to die to the sounds of palpitating whispers.

Discuss your surgical biopsy.

What brought you the most strength during the early days of your diagnosis?

Do you remember any of your dreams?

6 The Surgical Decision

"Make it a rule of life never to regret and never look back. We all live in suspense, from day to day, from hour to hour; in other words, we are the hero of our own story."

—Mary McCarthy

My reading on the Internet and in medical textbooks taught me that DCIS is rarely fatal and this brought me some comfort. .The books I read each day suggested that the prognosis was good. Although there was a slim chance that at a later date, DCIS could show up in the other breast.

My nights became painful episodes of tossing and turning. Our king-sized bed seemed smaller than usual. I felt trapped within myself and trapped within my mind's roaming thoughts. The nighttime demons would not leave me alone. So a few days after speaking with Dr. Silverstein, I drove to the bookstore and strolled up and down the self-help section. A book by Louise Hay called *You Can Heal Your Life* caught my eye. I plopped down on the plush sofa near the stairwell of Barnes and Noble and read Hay's thoughts on the causes of cancer. She believed one of the contributory reasons for cancer is a result of a hurt and long-standing resentment, deep secrets of grief that eat away at the self.

As a nurse, I understand that all health conditions are caused by a complex interaction of multiple causes and that there is not one reason for a cancer diagnosis. Cancer could be the result of viral infections, carcinogenic chemicals in our environment, or perhaps from sun exposure during childhood and/or long-term stress that can interfere with immune system functioning. But I meditated on the possibility that there was sadness burrowed inside me. I wondered about the deep trauma from finding my grandmother dead when I was only ten years old, and how that incident, still so vivid in my mind, had scarred some part of me.

I began thinking about my relationship with my mother.

I had already read Vivian Gornick's *Fierce Attachments* and related so much to her words and to her relationship with her own mother. She says, "Her pain [her mother's] became my element, the country in which I lived, the rule beneath which I bowed. It commanded me, made me respond against my will. I longed endlessly to get away from her."

I reflected upon how often as a child I had sensed being in my mother's way and how she would rather be horseback riding than be with me. Before my father died, he'd said, "You know your mother didn't want any children. When we spoke about starting a family she said that all she wanted was a parakeet." My father spent months trying to convince her that a life without children is no life at all. He told me his desire to have children was magnified by losing most of his family in the Holocaust after he himself had spent five of his formative years in the Dachau concentration camp.

Reading Hay's book gave me a passport into understanding the sadness that for years had been buried in my soul. It also gave me permission to grieve about certain aspects of my past and empowered me to mourn. I felt the hidden gorge from past pains now widening inside of me. I carefully put the binoculars on my childhood and acknowledged some deep-seated complaints and concerns. My cancer diagnosis became a stir-fry of emotions cooking inside me. The pan was simmering and I could not shut off the burner.

Tapping into my past made the cancer seem larger. I flip-flopped back and forth from being afraid of the surgery to wanting it as quickly as possible. For the most part, I wanted the cancer yanked out of me. I had confidence that I would be in the hands of one of the country's best breast surgeons and I did not want to waste any time seeking more opinions.

My surgery was scheduled for August 21st. On August 19th, both my daughters would celebrate their birthday. Rachel would turn eighteen and Regine sixteen. Way before my scheduled surgery, they had planned a joint backyard birthday party with all of their friends. The homemade invitations had been sent out, the food was ordered and the entertainment arranged. Simon suggested the party be cancelled. My gut told me this is what I would have done if my mother was scheduled to have surgery a few days later. Yet, another part of me wanted my girls to carry on with their plans.

A week before my operation, over dinner, we discussed my surgery. I could see in both my daughters' eyes that they were torn. For months their project had been the planning of this party together, and they were proud to have done it on their own, with little assistance from us. But I could see they now questioned how they could be celebrating the day before their mother was flying to California for major surgery.

I was incapable of helping in their decision. I had my own issues and decisions to make, so all I said was that if they decided to proceed with the party, they should not expect me to mingle with their friends like I would normally do. (I had no desire to talk and make jokes with fifty teenagers. It was difficult enough staying clear of my tissue box.) I knew my emotions would boil over, especially while watching my beautiful daughters blow out their birthday candles. While we were all still mulling over the situation, my wonderful father-in-law phoned and said, "I think the girls should continue with their plans. They need to celebrate their birthday."

At the time I was disappointed, but now I believe he guided us correctly, as he had done many times before and since. My own father often said: "In the Jewish religion, if there is a happy and a sad event on the same day, like a wedding and a funeral and you don't know which to attend, always go to the happy one."

The days before I had to leave for California for the surgery were some of the most agonizing of my life. Similar to the week my father died, I could not stop crying. Buckets of tears poured out of me. My mouth was continuously parched and my family had to ensure that I remained hydrated. I barely slept, and for the first time in my life I sought the assistance of sleeping pills. Darkness fell upon my soul in every imaginable way. I meditated about my past, present, and future.

I became a prisoner to my own thoughts.

Other than my journal, the thing that helped me the most was my portable CD player, for which I bought a slew of new age compact discs at the alternative health store. After sprinkling lavender oil on my pillow and body, I lay down to listen to the relaxing music. Each night before bed, I stirred a few tablespoons of honey into a cup of milk and then warmed it in the microwave. Other times, chamomile tea or a glass of red wine worked just fine. I held tightly onto Simon while he slept soundly.

During this agonizing time, I also had numerous telephone conversations with the plastic surgeon, and his nurse. There was so much information to digest and so much to decide. It would have been much easier buying a car. I devoured *Dr. Susan Love's Breast Book*. It provided all the answers and explanations any woman could possibly want. My plastic surgeon's nurse sent me a twenty-page facsimile explaining all my reconstruction options. I learned that most women opt for the expander method of reconstruction. In this type of surgery, a hollow sack is placed behind the chest muscle and everything is sewn closed. A little tube and valve is attached to the sac, and over the course of three to six months, the surgeon injects increasing amounts of saline solution until the sac is completely full. When the sac reaches the desired size, the tube is removed. But this procedure was not a viable option for me, because there was no surgeon in Orlando willing to perform the weekly inflations (particularly since I had chosen a Californian surgeon to do the mastectomy and reconstruction all at one time.)

My plastic surgeon specialized in a reconstruction called the *latissimus dorsi* myocutaneous flap. It involves moving a flap of fat, muscle, and skin from the back (on the same side as the mastectomy.) The skin and underlying fat remain connected to the muscle, and the muscle (with its own blood supply) is tunneled under the skin (just before the armpit) into the hole that has been created in the breast by the mastectomy. The muscle is then repositioned in the breast to create a sort of a hammock to hold a saline implant.

I read all the pages of the facsimile and phoned the nurse with my medical history questions.

"I spoke with the doctor," she said. "He believes strongly in your having the *latissimus dorsi* flap surgery. This is his specialty. He says it's a one-step operation where you don't have to come to the office for repeated office visits like the other option. He's had a lot of success with this type of surgery."

On paper, the surgery looked intimidating and frightful. It seemed as if my entire upper torso would be completely transformed. Even though I would still be under anesthesia, having the *latissimus dorsi* reconstruction after a mastectomy would be akin to two major surgeries. And the recovery would be much longer, painful and more complicated. I already knew from past cesareans and my breast biopsies that my body was not good at healing.

I felt I had no other viable choice, though, so I opted for this surgery. I never thought about my history of muscular aches and pains. Everyone has their vulnerable body parts, which flare-up under stress. My father-in-law, for example, gets stomachaches when he is upset, and my mother-in-law gets migraines. I manifest stress in the muscles of my upper body, particularly my neck and shoulders. Only years later would I realize how much my body suffered from losing this muscle segment from my mid-back. To this day there is a continuous tightening in the area and often, without warning, the muscle becomes even tighter. (After a year or so I hired a trainer who has helped me rebuild my muscle structure.)

Looking back on the decision, it would have been a better idea to be more aggressive in finding a local surgeon who could follow me post-operatively, so that I could have chosen the expander method of breast reconstruction. I have learned that in the long run it has fewer complications post-operatively.

In the end, I would wind up with two rather large incisions, one on my breast, and the other in the middle of my back under my bra strap. Yet I would also get both surgeries done at the same time. So I would wake up with a mound on my chest in the same spot where my breast had been removed.

Life Handed Me a Memoir

Only a year after father found her—
the parakeet she wanted instead of a kid,
my mother gave birth to me

on Mother's Day in the middle
of last century, making me more than
halfway to being an octogenarian.

Now that she's almost a century old,
my mother realizes a girl bird couldn't care
for her aged needs—nursing, bathing, meals.

I take flights across the country
so the little woman she
never wanted can embrace her.

I am okay with all of this
because it's given me plenty
of fodder to write about,

plus my father is looking down
at me smiling at what
a blessing Mother's Day has became.

Did you reach for any books that helped you either during your pre-surgical or post-surgical time?

What book or person helped you the most in understanding what you were going through?

Did you have a choice between having a mastectomy or lumpectomy? If so, what were your feelings about your choice and the decision you made?

What treatment was recommended for you? What were your options and what were the advantages and disadvantages of each?

7   The Surgery

"You gain strength, courage and confidence by every experience in which you really stop to look fear in the face... You must do the thing which you think you cannot do."

—Eleanor Roosevelt

On August 20th, the day after my daughters' birthday party, Simon and I checked into our hotel in California. .For the next few weeks we would call that place our home. Prior to this surgery, I had flipped into survival mode in order to psychologically prepare myself for what was to come—if that was possible. Whether the house was tidy or whether my attire was suitable for grocery shopping became insignificant. I taught myself not to sweat the small things. Although normally a good listener, my skills dwindled as I became tangled up in the whirlwind of my own issues and illness. Simon found himself having to repeat everything to me. My concentration was gridlocked, but his positive attitude often helped to swing me back into focus. He reminded me over and over again how lucky we were to catch the cancer early. And while it was nice hearing his compassionate words, the truth is they provided a minuscule amount of comfort, for there was pain burrowing a hole deep inside me.

On the morning of my third journey to The USC Norris Cancer Hospital—the morning that would ultimately change my life forever, I held my right breast and thanked it for all of the joy and pleasure it had brought into my life. I said I was sorry to have to say good-bye. I never wanted my daughters to have to go through any of this. I pleaded with my deceased dad to see to it that in their lifetime, someone would find a cure for all types of cancer.

The following hours of pre-operative chaos in the hospital passed in a blur: X-rays, blood tests and more mammograms. In spite of a double dose of sleeping pills the night before, I had difficulty falling asleep knowing that the following day I would lose my breast forever. The fog still had not lifted. While the rest of the teaching hospital lined up outside the cafeteria for lunch, I was being checked into the pre-operative holding area. For the last time, I put a gown over two whole breasts. I looked down and took a deep breath, longing for it to be over. The wait was killing me. Each time the curtains were drawn around me for another test, I prayed it would be the last. Finally, the senior nurse inserted an intravenous needle into the bulging vein inside my left elbow. *Thank goodness!* That needle would free me from my thoughts. Simon gave me the tightest hug imaginable and told me that he would be waiting outside. My foggy head began feeling heavy as they wheeled me through the double doors into a very cold room.

Bifurcation

Having a breast sliced off
leaves a woman with two lives—
the one before the loss
and the one after.

To My Daughters

You were the first I thought of
when diagnosed with what
strikes one in eight women.

It was too soon to leave you,
but I thought it a good sign
that none of us were born

under its pestilent zodiac.
I stared at the stars and wished
upon each one that you'd never

wake up as I did this morning
to one real breast and one fake one;
but that the memories you carry

will be only sweet ones, and then
I remembered you had your early traumas
of being born too soon, and losing

a beloved grandpa too young. I have
this urge to show you the scars
on the same breasts you both cuddled

as babies, but then I wonder why
you'd want to see my imperfections
and perhaps your destiny. I cave in

and show you anyway, hoping you learn
to eat well and visit your doctors, but then

I wonder if it really matters, as I remember

what your grandpa Umpie used to say,
"When your time's up, it's up."
May he always watch over you!

During this time, did you or anyone else notice any unusual
personality changes?

Describe your admission to the hospital.

What are some of the questions you asked or would like to ask?

8   Post-Surgical Notes

"The psychic scars caused by believing that you are ugly leave a permanent mark on your personality."

—Joan Rivers

The first four days following surgery remain a blur. I do remember .Simon trying everything to soothe my crying eyes. I also recall being in a private room with flowers lining the windowsill and my favorite one was the white *phalaenopsis* orchid that outlasted all the other flowers. I remember a big stack of used tissues on my bedside table—evidence of my uncontrollable tears. I recall Simon bringing me three beanie babies, which was the craze at the time, each one representing one of my three kids. I remember the first evening after my surgery, and how Simon pulled out his digital camera (not yet as commonplace as they are today) to take photographs of me, and then sent them across the computer line back to our kids in Orlando. As an engineer, he is often one step ahead.

I really did not want my picture taken. I preferred not being seen looking like a car had run over me. But, Simon insisted it would bring the family solace, since they were more than 3,000 miles away. Simon was my Rock of Gibraltar in every sense of the word. I could never have survived without him. My other best friend was my journal. My daughter Rachel, knowing how particular I was about journals, knocked on my bedroom door just before I left for California. She kneeled beside me as I was sitting on the floor with my suitcase beside me. With her smile that lit up my room, she handed me a red and beige floral journal. I brought her close to me and squeezed her with all my might, and then she watched me tuck my new journal into a safe corner of my suitcase.

Immediately following surgery, I did not feel much like writing. All I wanted to do was sleep and cry, but somehow I managed a few paragraphs. Here are some of the thoughts written at that time. The first one is my first day post-op:

August 22, 2001

I wake up in the Intensive Care Unit (ICU) today and Simon sits beside me holding my hand. One part of me wants to look down at the hospital gown covering this corset-like gauze bandage around my chest. Yet another part of me is scared out of my mind. The nurse helps me to the bathroom and I avoid the mirror as if it holds the most dreaded secret. I want to rip it off the bathroom wall. I never want to see myself naked. While walking back to bed, I glance towards the window begin sobbing with no respite. I know in my heart that one day soon I will have to look at my chest. My hope is that my plastic surgeon will make all the necessary explanations. I am happy that the surgery is behind me, but now I must begin preparing to walk down an even more arduous road. I must get used to the new me.

August 23, 2001

Today my mood oscillates back and forth. One moment I want to touch my newly-created breast and the next minute I never want to see it. I am pleased that the reconstruction was done immediately following the mastectomy while I was still under anesthesia. After breakfast, I pulled the nurse's cord for assistance to sit up. I am terribly sore from being in one position. By the time she arrives moments later, I have already changed my mind. I put my hand over my right breast and feel nothing. I do the same on the left. I can only feel the slight pressure of my hand. How will I ever get used to having no sensations? My right nipple had always been more sensitive and more easily stimulated than my left, but now there is a sense of nothingness, numbness, a void.

Today the nurse removed the bandage from around my chest. I looked the other way while crying into my pillow. I felt nothing. My plastic surgeon said some sensations might eventually return, but never again could I become sexually aroused by being touched on my right side. So, I have two breasts, but really only one. My sensations have been severed forever. Never again would I experience that sublime tingling when fingers run over my rather large nipple—never again on that side. Never could I experience the joy and tingles from the let-down reflex when my babies sucked for the first time. I loved that sensation which permeated my soul and brought me such joy.

August 27, 2001

The books I have read and my nursing experience warned me that depression is common following many surgeries, particularly breast surgery, because of the huge psychological component of losing a breast. I should be optimistic because Dr. Silverstein says that the cancer has been removed. He believes I am lucky that the cancer did not spread into my lymph nodes. Yes, this is a true blessing, but there are moments when this is not simply enough to console me. My father taught me to look at the glass half full and not half empty. I'm trying. Really trying. But, this entire event has been surreal. My defenses are stripped. I have no strength left in my body except for the weeping. Tears flow like an endless river. They pour out without warning and dry up without notice.

August 28, 2001

I look around and see all the technology. I think of my husband, an engineer, and how people like him have made so many people's survival possible. He is a fixer. As on so many other occasions, he wants to quickly make everything better for me. His smile and touch are healing, but even with all his power, he cannot bring my breast back to me. If only someone had a magical wand to make me feel better. Simon implores me to think positively.

Sometimes life is not so simple. It's still early in my post-operative period, but I already feel physically and emotionally changed and drained. In some ways it is easier being far from home. My predicament somehow seems clearer and my mind less distracted by these unfamiliar surroundings.

September 3, 2001

Today I am nearly two weeks post-op. I do not feel any better emotionally than the day they rolled me out of the cold and sterile operating room. My emotional strength is barely returning. I still get teary-eyed for no obvious reason. This morning, the nurses bathed me. They helped me to the chair where I tried to read a magazine, but my mind wanders. Everything makes me cry, even glancing at the latest hairstyles in the magazines. I feel trapped inside this body which I no longer know.

Here's what I look like: On my right side is a drainage tube tucked into a hole beneath my mastectomy site. On the same side, another tube leads to the incision in my back where they have removed the muscle and tissue to cup my saline implants. The tube leads to this thing that looks like a hand grenade which dangles from my side. This grenade drains the blood from my wounds, but I think it does the same from my heart. It needs to be emptied three times each day. It's gross, and yet another reminder of my missing breast. When we go to dinner at the hotel's restaurant, the only thing I can wear are baggy men's shirts to hide my tube and stupid grenade.

Getting up and going to the bathroom is such an ordeal. I need at least ten minutes to prepare for the departure from my bed. Getting all the wires organized is truly a monumental task. I cannot lean on my back; the drainage tube sticks straight out. I cannot lean on my right side—another tube. They hurt like hell. There are no more comfortable positions left for me. Jeannine [mother-in-law] asked if I have been writing. She must be kidding! I have so much to write about, but I cannot focus. My mind wanders beyond belief. Life is fuzzy and not even eyeglasses can help. I am just plain frustrated. I can only muster these few words, which alone drain me of all of my energy.

September 4, 2001

I went to see my plastic surgeon today and he said I was not ready to travel back home to Orlando. He removed the mastectomy drain, but said that there was still lots of fluid coming from the drainage tube in my back incision. He admits that it is more drainage than he originally anticipated. I am deeply disappointed. I fiercely miss my kids. I'm trying to relax and recover and take

*daily walks around the nearby flower gardens. The sitting
area in my room has many flowers and on the coffee table
is a huge box of chocolate turtles from sent by husband's
cousins. Chocolate is a wonderful panacea for the blues. I
am sick and tired of crying.*

*It seems as if the past couple of weeks have been
surreal. A thick cloud suspends over me. How did I get
here? I was diligent about my annual mammograms and
check-ups. On the first day of my menstrual cycle, I
religiously did self-breast exams in the shower. There is
no cancer in my family. Why am I lying here all
mutilated?*

*I have never thought much about cancer, but one thing
I know is that if cancer is in your body, you better get it
out quickly.*

*Having had reconstructive surgery at the same time as
my mastectomy has put my mind at ease. Even though I
have refrained from looking at myself naked in the
mirror, there was a sense of relief to waking up with a
mound on my right side, even if it was not my very own
breast, but just a sack of saline water.*

September 6, 2001

*Prior to my surgery, I scanned books and articles about
my type of breast cancer and what to expect after surgery.
I read in my bathroom, in carpool lines, and in bed before
the sleeping pills kicked in. Most of the time, I wanted to
know everything, yet there were times when I wanted to
know absolutely nothing. Sometimes ignorance is bliss.
Simon, on the other hand, wanted to know everything
about everything. It was probably the scientist in him
craving all the details of what to expect during the surgery
and the post-operative period. Today I am petrified of
details. I was never a textbook case, even with my high-*

risk pregnancies laden with bed rest, so why should this time be different?

I'm trying to take the position that cancer is no longer lurking inside me. I did have cancer, but it is now all gone. All of it. I really don't like the sound of the term 'breast cancer.' People equate cancer with death. I refuse to die, but just in case I do, I have to write a poem for my family. Here it is:

Message to My Family

The day after I die
and hours after my ashes cool,
find a purple urn with a window.

Purple nurtures my spiritual strength
and windows keep me alive. Remember
I'm claustrophobic and the thought

of being stuck inside a box frightens me,
since I must indulge in my favorite hobby
of people-watching, which sends me

to my journal where I find joy and solace.
Remember, writers need time alone—
once a day my window should be closed,

just once a day after I die.

When I first learned about my breast cancer, I wanted to hear everybody else's escapades and medical sagas. It seems as if everyone knows someone who has had breast cancer. Listening to other people's stories is boring at times, and at other times scary. Sometimes it is inspiring to learn that others are less fortunate than I. The woman in the corridor told me about her Stage III cancer. Okay, she made me feel lucky, but I just don't want to be surrounded by negative energy.

I am so afraid that the cancer will come back. I cry about losing the breast and also about having to lose my other one. Crying comes so easily. Sometimes the tears last a few minutes, other times an hour. It all depends.

September 7, 2001

Today Simon asked me why I was crying. Men don't always understand these things. It must be a Venus and Mars thing. He thought I should be happy because the surgery was all behind me. He is impatient for me to feel better. I think I need to talk to other women. I phoned my friend in California who'd had cancer four years ago. She connected me with a support group called, WIN ABC (Women's Information Network Against Breast Cancer). I phoned and told them about my surgery. Two days later a group of ladies visited my hotel room to perform a ritualistic healing circle. It was incredible. They lined chairs up around the small coffee table. At the end, they placed the large armchair for me. Simon sat beside me.

One lady wrapped a protective wool shawl around my shoulders. Another lady lit candles on the coffee table. We all held hands as they sang and prayed for me. I did not understand a word because they sang in Hebrew, but the melodies were soothing. The room became a Mecca of positive healing energy. During the ceremony I cried a lot.

At one point my tears turned into sobs. Simon leaned over and said, shhhh. The lady on the other side of him leaned over and told him that it was okay for me to cry. (Another Venus and Mars thing.) At the end of the ceremony the ladies all gathered around me and one at a time gave me a hug. The event loosened my emotions like cupping loosens secretions from a congested lung. I cried even harder after the women left. Simon took my hand in his and told me how beautiful I was and consoled me as best as he could.

On my twelfth day post-op I went for yet another appointment with my plastic surgeon.

"Well, Diana, I think you'll be happy with the news I'm about to give you," he said, standing in front of me with his hands on my shoulders. "Your drain is ready to be removed." I moved closer and gave him a hug. I could not have been happier. It would have been impossible to bear yet another day wearing baggy shirts to hide my grenade. Plus, I was so sick and tired of hotels and hotel food. I was dying to see my kids, and no matter how many photos Simon had posted of them, it was not enough to encircle me with their love and radiant smiles.

We arrived at the airport and checked our bags. I walked slowly beside Simon through the terminal. My pillow cupped my chest for support and protection. It also helped set up a barrier between me and the rest of the world. I detected the way people stared at me, wondering what had happened. I was delighted that no one asked about my indelible experience. They could have run the risk of a pillow being flung in their face. An unusual bubbling of anger began surfacing within me—all the aftermath of gallons of anesthesia, and the shock of the events of the past two weeks.

Robbed Twice

The day after the doctor
cut off my breast
I got on the phone
to my therapist
who told me to give
myself some time
to figure out who I am
after being slashed
by the knife.

What do you remember about the first few days following your surgery?

What pathology reports did you receive?

If you are having chemotherapy, describe how you are feeling. What side effects are you having?

How long did you have to stay in the hospital? What did you think when your doctor said that you were ready to go home?

9 Recovery and 9/11

"We don't see things as they are; we see them as we are."
— Anaïs Nin

On September 10th, 2001, my friend Loren phoned to wish Simon a happy birthday. She then asked to speak to me. .

"Diana, how are you feeling, my love?"

"Still weak, but getting stronger each day."

"I wondered if you thought you were ready for visitors?" she asked.

"Not really, but, you yes."

Initially, I really did not want any visitors, but because she was a nurse, Loren would be compassionate and know what to say and how to say it. I thought she might also know when it was time to leave to give me time to rest, so I decided her visit would be okay.

"How about I come tomorrow morning about ten o'clock and bring bagels?"

"Great. I am looking forward to it," I said.

Although I had told Loren it was okay to visit, as soon as I hung up the phone, I had mixed feelings. I wanted to see her, but I was still so self-conscious about my appearance. I was also concerned about how labile my emotions were and the possibility of crying from the moment she walked in until the moment she left. The plan was for her to arrive at ten o'clock on the morning of September 11th, 2001. At eight-fifty she phoned sounding absolutely frantic.

"Are you watching the news? Did you see what happened? I'm beside myself. Are you near your television? You just won't believe it!"

Loren's daughter and my son were in the entertainment industry so I thought she wanted me to see the reviews of a newly released show or movie. I could never have imagined what I saw before my eyes. A plane had crashed into one of the World Trade Centers in New York. I gasped in disbelief and horror. Almost one hour later at 9:40 a.m., another plane crashed into the second tower and it too went crashing to the ground. I grasped my incisions and phoned Simon at work.

For the first week, this horrific event encircled my isolated world spanning from my bedroom to the family room. In a sad way, the horrors distracted me from my own healing woes, but they also magnified my feelings of despair and sadness. I became increasingly emotional while watching the city of my youth being torn apart and shook up like never before. The tears surged out of me. Below are some of my journal entries:

September 18, 2001

Even after a week since the Twin Towers came tumbling down, I remain glued to the television screen. What else is there to do at home all day long? I cannot concentrate on reading, and my writing is not flowing. Like many other Americans I realize that watching television is highly addictive. We sit trying to make some sense of the happenings and try to understand what type of monsters could do such a terrible thing. They suspect terrorism. I grieve for my city's loss while grieving for the loss of my breast. My emotions are so overwhelming that I want to put a pillow over my face and call it quits.

Drinking calming tea in the morning and drinking chardonnay at night is helping me cope with all this anxiety.

During the weeks following my surgery, I pondered the other losses in my life and how I had handled them. Emotions about my city and my breast cancer became intertwined. My mind turned into a fast-paced movie. Helplessness watered my world. Nothing I could do would bring back my breast or the World Trade Center. I felt like a helpless observer in a world quickly passing me by.

It seemed as if all the reasons for sadness rushed to the surface. I was unable to see any goodness around me. It became a struggle to laugh at my husband's jokes. I became depressing to be around. Yet in spite of all these symptoms I fought the diagnosis of depression. I was petrified of falling into the dark pits and fought it with all of my might. I did not want to announce defeat to my cancer nor to depression. I wanted to survive like my grandmother had survived the First World War...though in the end, the hauntings of her youth and many years of depression led to her demise. I repeatedly thought about my grandmother and the sense of loss I felt when she took her life forty years earlier. I reminisced about all the special moments we shared for the first ten years of my life when she was my primary caretaker. The pain of losing her became more intense with every passing year. I was too young to die and had too much to live for.

A few days after 9/11, Simon and I decided that it was best for me to shut off the television during the day. The sad news about the people who had died coupled with the sadness of the families left behind just compounded my own personal pain. Emotionally, I was not strong enough to handle it all.

When Simon came home at night we turned the television back on. This ritual minimized my sense of despair. During the day, I nurtured my favorite old habits of reading and writing to generate my strength.

September 29, 2001

Five weeks have already passed since my surgery. In many ways it has gotten easier, but in other ways I am still battling with accepting my loss. I find myself asking many questions. Did I make the right decision? Should I have gone for more opinions? What if I had had my mammogram earlier?

My thoughts have become more and more profound. I no longer fight the mask of depression. I still have trouble accepting the fact that I had cancer. I wondered how they knew for sure that no more cancer cells lurk somewhere else in my body. I am petrified.

During my healing period, I needed loving care from everyone who crossed my path. It was around this time when I had an appointment for a dental cleaning. The hygienist was rough while cleaning my teeth, and she was *not* tenderhearted. Before beginning, she plunked her instruments right on top of my surgical site. One poked through the little paper bib slung around my neck. I asked her to be careful and not put the instruments there, and she gave me this dirty look as if to say, "don't tell me how to do my job."

Tears formed in my eyes as I battled with the embarrassment of telling her that she laid her stuff on my newly created breast and surgical site. I ended up speaking privately with the dentist whom I had known for more than fifteen years and he promised me that he would speak to her. It was at that point when I realized that it is best to be honest and forthright with people, rather than suffering in silence.

October 1, 2001

These have been some of the worst months of my life. So many times, I wanted to step outside my body and live in someone else's. I wanted to walk in someone else's shoes for a minute, an hour or even a day. I am deeply exhausted, both emotionally and physically. I want the pain to dissolve like the peppermint resting on my tongue. Simon says I am moody, but how could I not be? One day I am so happy to be alive, and the next day all I want to do is curl up and call it quits.

I'm caught between the confusion and the strangulation of my thoughts concerning my future and the images from my past. I badly want to be alive to see my children get married and become parents themselves, but I am petrified that I won't live that long. Are the doctors telling me the truth? Maybe they don't want to upset me. Maybe my prognosis is not so good. I yearn to one day rock my grandchildren in my arms, smell sweet formula on their breath and change an unbearably stinky diaper. How frustrating it is to have such little control over my own destiny!

To Dettner (My grandmother)

You took your life in the house where
we lived together forty years ago.
I was ten and you sixty.
Your ashen face and blonde bob
disheveled upon white sheets

on the stretcher held by paramedics
lightly grasping each end, and tiptoeing

down the creaking wooden stairs
you walked up the night before.

But now your body descended to the ambulance
and sirens swarmed like vultures

around the place I once called home.
I wonder why you left in such a way,

as the depression gnawed
at your gentle heart, which cared for me

since my very first push into the world.
I've learned from you

never to give up, but to find
a passion and thank you

I did.
I live to write
so I shall never die.

Did any event, personal or in the current affairs, affect your physical or emotional healing?

How did you feel about being at home?

10 Follow-up

"The things we overcome in life become our strengths."
—Anne Bancroft

I continued to be followed in Orlando by the oncologist who referred me to Dr. Silverstein in Los Angeles. At my six-week check up, I felt ready to discuss the genetics of my disease. .

"Have you read *My Breast* by Joyce Wadler?" I asked.

"No, I haven't."

"It's a short book about her breast cancer story. At the end she speaks about how four years after having breast cancer she was diagnosed with ovarian cancer. It was a riveting and frightening story. She said that one in one hundred Ashkenazi Jews carry the *185delAG* mutation gene that predisposes women to both breast and ovarian cancer."

"And why did you find that interesting?" he inquired.

"I'm a Jew and my parents were from Eastern Europe."

"I didn't know you were Jewish." He continued, "In that case, let's order you to have genetic testing," He looked up at his nurse taking notes. "There's definitely a chance of a genetic factor here."

I did not want to tell him that Dr. Silverstein had already sent me for a consultation with a prominent oncologist in Los Angeles who after a two-hour session ascertained that I was at a low-risk for having the breast cancer gene. Although his was a thorough consultation based on a model of questions, as the mother of two daughters, I thought a blood test might also be a good idea.

"Truthfully," I said, "I don't know if I am psychologically ready for a blood test yet. I really can't take any more bad news right now."

"That's fine. There's no rush. Why don't we talk about it again in six months?" He nodded to his nurse.

"That sounds good to me," I said.

When six months rolled around his nurse phoned to remind me. She gave me all the details. She described the test as highly sophisticated and costing about three thousand dollars.

"It will take anywhere from three to six months to get approval from your insurance company," she said. I gave her the green light to begin the process.

As it turned out, the most tenuous aspect of having this test was waiting three long weeks for the results. The nurse said that if the results were positive, the doctor would phone me, if they were negative she would phone.

Three weeks after taking the test, I delighted in hearing the nurse's voice on the other end of the phone. She explained the results and reiterated that just because I did not have that particular gene did not mean my daughters and I were at no risk for breast cancer. She said our risk was the same as the rest of the general population. Back then the risk was one in eight for breast cancer, although today, for cancers overall, the risk is about one in three. I never reported my results to my daughters. I did not want the false confidence of not carrying the cancer gene to result in their neglecting to take care of their breasts and having regular exams. My oncologist recommended that their gynecologists should begin watching them closely in their late twenties. For my eldest daughter that would be only ten years away.

In October 2001, Simon and I prepared for our next trek out to California. There were two reasons for the trip. First, I would have the second part of my reconstructive surgery— not as big an ordeal as my last surgery, but surgery, nevertheless. This surgery was to construct a new nipple on the breast that was reconstructed in August. My plastic surgeon would use my surrounding breast tissue to create a newly formed nipple. Because I had no sensations on that side there would be no pain associated with this surgery. Second, my plan was to meet with a holistic internist, who came very highly recommended.

This physician, who now calls himself an integrative medical specialist, is a well-known practitioner and only sees patients based on personal referral. "You've got to see him," my cousin said. "He will help you. He's absolutely wonderful." She continued to rave about him and his medical sensibilities and how he had helped so many people. I was receptive and desperate to hear any advice that would steer me onto a healthy path. My nerves were strung out, primarily because since my surgery, no physician other than my breast surgeons had seen me naked. But I jotted down his phone number in my red cloth journal anyway, and phoned his office for an appointment and thought on this next visit out to California I would make an appointment with him.

The lush waiting room was on the third floor of a medical building with a big picture window overlooking the Los Angeles skyline. Because of this physician's high profile, I expected a waiting room packed with patients. What I found was the complete opposite. No other patients were there. To me this was an indication of a well-managed office. The room was light and airy, with two beige loveseats, a beige sofa, and calming wall hangings. A coffee table featured magazines protected by plastic sheaths, and in front of one of the loveseats was a foot massage machine. Naturally, I chose to sit there. New age music whispered in the background and at the reception window sat a pretty woman in her fifties wearing a crisp white turban. She lifted her head to acknowledge my presence. Working behind her were two other women wearing turbans who also gracefully acknowledged my arrival.

After checking in, I was told to have a seat. Only moments later a young and bright-eyed nurse holding my chart peeked into the waiting room through the glass door. She called my name and then walked me to the small, clean examination room with shelves of herbs and diagnostic machines. Before the physician's arrival, she asked me a few salient questions. She remained with me until he arrived, moments later. He extended his hand and gave me a firm handshake. Not only did this man's eyes emanate intelligence, they also pierced right through me. I sensed that even without knowing me, he knew my secrets.

"It's a pleasure to meet you. You have a wonderful cousin," he said, glancing down at my medical questionnaire, which indicated my cousin as the referral.

"Yes. She is."

"So tell me a little about your health," he said.

I gave him all the details and he did not waste any time dashing to the point.

"I wish I had met you before all that, but since I did not have that luxury, I will do my best to keep you healthy. How does that sound?" he asked.

A tear fell down my cheek. I never wanted cancer growing inside me ever again, and something about this man instilled a deep trust in me. After documenting more of my history, he told me that as my doctor, he would take care of me so that cancer would have only a slim chance of recurring. He also mentioned that he had patients who had flown in from all over the world to see him and that the geographical distance would not be a problem. He offered numerous recommendations, some to be shared on this visit and others on subsequent visits.

After an extensive physical examination, he ordered an array of blood tests. He recited the names of some herbs that his nurse jotted down on a yellow form with my prescribed dosage. After my appointment, they directed me up the corridor to the supplement department to get my order filled—an herbal pharmacy right within his office. Greeting me at the window was a friendly woman in her thirties who was to fill my order. Within ten minutes she had filled a medium-sized paper bag with a cornucopia of supplements. Included in the bag was also a bottle of white powder to be mixed with water that would neutralize my body's pH. My new physician believed that cancer cells prefer an acidic environment and he implored me to work on keeping my urine alkaline. This meant limiting my coffee and alcohol intake and eating lots of vegetables. Each morning I would monitor my urine pH with a little strip of paper and then mark it on a chart he sent home with me. If my urine was too acidic (5.0 or below) I would neutralize it by mixing that white powder with water and drinking it.

He also shared a few other helpful recommendations, such as incorporating spiritual or relaxing modalities into my lifestyle. He suggested Kundalini Yoga. This type of yoga balances the glandular system and strengthens the nervous system. Yoga, he also said, had the power to help us gain control over both our emotions and our minds. After arriving back home, my mission was to locate a convenient ashram. (I found a suitable one, and I drove there two or three times each week to practice meditation, breathing, and some light chanting. I always left feeling refreshed and rejuvenated. It is incredibly invigorating and relaxing.)

Also during that initial appointment, he provided the name of a psychotherapist and suggested we meet before my journey back to Orlando.

The next day, I met with my new therapist and she graciously and efficiently crammed her three-part appointment into one session. During our time together, she taught me how to do creative visualization for relaxation. At the end of the ninety-minute session, she gave me a large envelope. Inside was a specific protocol, some relaxation tapes and her phone number. She told me to call her if I had any questions. She also shared other tools for my psychological well-being. I was delighted to learn of her willingness to do phone sessions. Over the course of the following year, this woman became my lifeline, the person I phoned any time during the day or night. She became my confidant, friend and advocate, always with my best interest held close to her heart.

After the meeting with my psychotherapist, I trekked to the hospital for my surgery. He was right. This surgery was not as complicated as the one I had in August. He asked me to return to his office three days later before I was to return to Orlando.

October 8, 2001

Today I had my three-day post-operative appointment with my plastic surgeon. He told me that everything looked good. He then looked me deep in the eyes and asked how my writing was going.

"I really haven't written since before my surgery in August. I've had trouble focusing."

> *"I have a project for you," he said, smiling and exposing his perfectly aligned white teeth.*

My plastic surgeon has a busy practice and also travels the world doing smile surgery on less fortunate children for free. That is his true passion, bringing smiles across the faces of children who since birth were never able to smile. He does this surgery mainly on those living in third world countries. He enjoys bringing this pleasure to kids and their families. He told me that his only frustration is not being able to see those children again after the surgery.

His second passion is breast surgery and here he gets to see the results of his work. He has a beautiful smile to go with his forty-something body, and strong hands that made me feel safe with them holding a knife.

"I want you to write a journal for me. And then I want you to send it to me. That would be a good project for you," he said at the end of my office visit before I returned to Orlando.

I sat down on the edge of the examination table looking and feeling stunned. *How did this man know about me and my needs? Who gave him the camera to peek inside of my head?*

I was delighted by his request and his perception of this writer's needs. I told him that writers never turn down a writing assignment, like plastic surgeons never turn down challenging cases. After that appointment, we flew back to Orlando. My first journal entry was a letter to him written on the airplane back to Orlando. I continued to keep in touch with him and once home, I bought myself a journal that would capture all my sentiments related to being a breast cancer survivor.

Below is one of the letters I wrote to my plastic surgeon after my second surgery:

December 12, 2001

Dear Doctor:

   I was very depressed this past weekend. I just couldn't stop crying. Nothing in particular sparked it except that I detest this time of the year. It is the anniversary of my father's death. We were so close. I miss him dearly.

   But, you know, everything makes me cry lately. These days, even meditating does not help. I don't even feel like working out. I must be more patient with myself. You told me to give myself a year. I am so impatient and so very obsessed with all my losses.

Diana

His Piano

My son sits at his grand piano,
back erect, fingers in place
on the glistening white keys,
unstirred by the sounds
of lawn mowers, dogs barking,
and airplanes flying above.

I plop down on the green velour sofa
to listen, yet embarrassingly
don't recognize the tunes,
or the names of all those songs
he's created. I'm yanked
into my seventeen-year-old's world
as he fills the high-ceiling room with his magic.

Five songs later, he motions me to his stool,
smiles into my eyes and places my fingers
on the keys. They become paralyzed.
I don't want his spot. My ears are tone deaf,
and I cannot remember a note.
I tell him I'd rather listen.

I return to the sofa, where I sit like a sponge
and a faucet at the same time. My tears
hold me hostage as my son's music soothes
my nerves. How will I ever thank him
for the joy he's brought into my middle-aged life
and the perfect posture I pestered him with as a child?

Java Genetics

Some look to their full-leafed
family tree for maps of

who they will become,
roadways to undiscovered selves.

While others glance at their parts
wondering where the mold

that formed them came from.
On some days, questions of beginnings

pour from my coffee-stained brain.
My answers are buried deeply

in the cemeteries of foreign lands
where mothers died during labor.

Were there any surprises following your surgery?

Do you think that you took care of yourself both physically and mentally prior to your diagnosis with breast cancer?

Did you decide to make any changes in your lifestyle following your diagnosis with breast cancer? If yes, what?

Did you find it necessary to see a therapist to help you cope?
If yes, describe that person and your relationship.

11   More Surgery

"Believing in yourself and liking yourself is all a part of good looks."

—Shirley Lord

In early February 2002, I was once again admitted to the Norris Hospital for my second—but completely elective reconstructive surgery. .This surgery was called maxoplexy, and was done on my normal breast. The idea was to lift it to match my newly created one. After having and nursing three kids, my breasts were understandably droopy. Even though it was not a part of my initial plan, my plastic surgeon convinced me that it would be a good idea to do this surgery because he suggested that down the road it would help me psychologically.

"You'll have a small incision under the breast in the crease, so you won't see it anyway. Then I'll put another incision around the areola. That's all," he added, making it sound so very easy, so matter-of-fact.

Whether it was my vanity at that moment, the good-looking plastic surgeon, or my husband sitting there saying, "do it, do it," or possibly a combination of all three; I consented to this additional elective surgery. While in California, I decided to also have a tattoo put on my newly reconstructed right breast.

The office of the nurse who did the tattoos was near my plastic surgeon's office. The rather short, dark-skinned lady called me in. There was nothing warm and fuzzy about her. She had a rushed and robotic way about her; I was just another case. For her this was a job and that was all. She closed the door and told me to lie down on the examination table. I unbuttoned my blouse and did so.

While wandering around the room looking for her tools, she said, "So you had a mastectomy?"

"Yes," I said curtly, but I almost said, "Why the hell else would I be here?"

She removed her color wheel from her tattoo box and brought it up to my breast to match the areola color of my left breast.

From her workstation, she got a bowl and mixed two colors together to find the perfect tint match. When she finally established the correct color, she poured it into the spout of this instrument resembling a pencil with nine fine needles at its tip, closely aligned beside one another.

As the tattooing process was about to begin my eyes began watering. I wanted it to be over. I did not want to think about my breasts anymore. I was sick of all the focus on them. I craved getting back to a normal life and the things I liked to do. As soon as she touched my breast with the color wheel, my eyes were completely clouded with tears. Feeling like she should say something, she quickly glanced at my face and then back to her work and said, "You're lucky not to have any sensations on your right side because tattooing can be quite painful."

Did she realize the real reason for my tears? I had just lost a breast! And not only that, I had no sensations whatsoever. For a sensual person like me, this was a huge loss. I felt very uncomfortable under the hand of this woman; she was either oblivious to my feelings or she had performed one too many of these procedures. I felt like suggesting she find another job;

burnout is not a good thing for someone in her position. However, I was thrilled to learn that the tattooing really did not hurt, although once in a while I had this radiating and tingling sensation dashing down the right side of my body.

February 5, 2002

Yesterday I had my second surgery in two months. The only difference this time around was that it was elective. I cannot believe that I actually chose to go through this hell! Honestly, the tips of too many surgical knives have butchered this body, once nestled in femininity. Never again will my body be the same. After this escapade, I see myself as a composite of a misplaced muscle and two flabby saline envelopes. This morning I had my normal boob lifted, and I ask, "Did I make the right decision?"

February 12, 2002

I glance in the bathroom mirror and see on my left side another battlefield, a trail of surgeon's knives. Did it really matter if I had one sagging breast and one perky one? Simon continuously reminds me of my beauty. Is he blind? Whom did I do this for? Anyway, am I supposed to look perfect at the age of forty-seven after having had three children and endured all the surgeries I have had?

I am dripping in grief. The pain in my left breast becomes worse at night when I lie down to sleep. With the first surgery I only felt pain in my back where the muscle was removed. This time it's different. I have become addicted to sleeping pills and soft-playing bedtime music. All that my mind wants to do is to wander deeper into the fields of sadness. Simon reminds me of all my blessings, but still I lie in bed with my eyes wet and closed. At times I force them to remain shut to block out the world, in the same way I forced my kids to eat spinach when they were little.

February 19, 2002

Dear Doctor:

I feel quite good today. I want to thank you for nudging me back into my writing haven. I haven't written seriously in months and maybe this has contributed to my depression. Writing always makes me feel better because I share my thoughts and that is why it is my best anti-depressant.

Yesterday I had a huge scare. With my left hand, I opened the car door and suddenly felt a muscle bulge in my chest. I froze in the middle of the street with the door still swung open as traffic buzzed by. I was too petrified to move. Phoning you crossed my mind, but it would have been six o'clock in the morning your time, plus I sensed that you would tell me that everything is probably okay.

My moods continue to fluctuate. Last week I was pissed off at myself for consenting to the elective surgery on my left side. I thought it might have been more gracious to be thankful for my life by leaving my body alone.

I just cannot depart from this state of recovery. I cannot lie on either my right or left side. It hurts no matter how I move. The new implant on the left side feels as if it will erupt from my skin. The skin is so taut around it. You promised me that it will loosen with time. I feel like a waterbed—afraid of being pricked by needles or the claws of my domestic animals. While running to his room yesterday, my son crashed into me. I stopped and touched my shirt, certain that it would be saturated with saline, but it wasn't. I just do not know how much impact these saline sacks can take.

For two weeks now, I have worn loose-fitting blouses. I am so self-conscious that people will notice how uneven my breasts are. My husband reminds me that most women do not have breasts the same size on both sides. I tossed all my old bras, v-necks and tight fitting sweaters into the Goodwill bag in the garage. On my last visit to California, you said I looked great. You stood in front of me with both your hands on my shoulders and said that I should wear more provocative clothes. You encouraged me to wear halters around the house and to get used to the new me. I bought a tight-fitting sweater. You know what? It felt great wearing it during our evening out.

Thank you for putting my mind, soul and body at ease. I can see why women fall in love with their plastic surgeons. Until next time, I remain your obliging patient,

Diana

February 20, 2002

Dear Doctor:

Thank you for spending time with me during my last visit to California. Your support has given me so much strength. I was so scared to have that surgery, but I'm glad it all worked out and that you convinced me that it was the right way to go.

Diana

Losing My Menopause

This morning a friend called to see if I'd gotten her card inviting me to the party, but I said that I did not and then told her I remembered that it had fallen out from the back pocket of my jeans into the toilet and yes, I will surely come and I apologized and said I must be losing my menopause but what I meant to say was that I was losing my mind but unfortunately not my extra weight. I think she understood.

Did you find that your moods fluctuated following your surgery? If yes, how did you handle your emotional issues?

Did you need subsequent surgeries or treatments, such as chemotherapy, radiation or tamoxifen? Describe.

Describe your experience the first time you went for treatments. What were you thinking?

What reoccurring thoughts do you have when you are having your treatments?

How do you feel about the medical staff and their attitude
when you go for treatments?

Describe how you feel when you are undressing and looking at yourself.

12 Emotional Reflections

"One of the things I learned the hard way was that it doesn't pay to get discouraged. Keeping yourself busy and making optimism a way of life can restore your faith in yourself."

— Lucille Ball

In the years after my initial breast cancer diagnosis, my emotions were like a rollercoaster. .I passed through so many shades of blue, rose and gray. I cried for the silliest reasons, such as when my artichokes burned on the stove or when my new puppy had been difficult to housetrain. Mostly, my tears were for inconsequential reasons. I felt more vulnerable than at any other time in my life. (And being pre-menopausal did not help my predicament.)

In a crazy sort of way, the amputation served as a gateway into my unconscious, and writing helped purge what had been bothering me at a deeper level. Some days my insights poured out directly onto my keyboard or into my journal and pages became flooded with words. But, on other days, I just wanted to move on with my life and forget about rehashing the issues of my past.

During the first year following my surgery, I held onto a lot of anger and frequently exploded at anyone who displayed the slightest negative attitude. The surgery left me with a sense of bitterness and the tendency to ruminate and ask questions, such as *why me?* I wanted people to feel sorry for me and understand what I had been through. I never thought of myself as a martyr, but I had the impulse to want to bathe in the world's sympathy. On good days, my positive side shined through and I expressed exuberance and appreciation for my life and embarrassment about my bouts with depression.

My family became my pillar of strength. Simon pulled me out of the depressive dungeons by reminding me of all I had to be thankful for. Even though I frequently felt stripped of the essence of being a woman, he continuously embraced my heart and my breasts, reminding me of my grandeur. My kids, Rachel, Regine and Joshua have always been so loving and tender with me and continued to make me feel appreciated, cherished and adored. It terrified me to think what their lives would be without me.

Sometimes looking on the bright side of things is a mechanism for obscuring realities that might be dangerous or threatening; with this in mind I continued to read articles and books proclaiming that there is a cancer personality. I reread Louise Hay's book, *You Can Heal Your Life* and through her words, tried to convince myself of my worthiness. I typed out this section and posted it beside my bed:

We are each responsible for all of our experiences.
Every thought we think is creating our future.
The point of power is always in the present moment.
Everyone suffers from self-hatred and guilt.
The bottom line for everyone is,
"I'm not good enough."

It's only a thought, and a thought can be changed.
We create every so-called illness in our body.

Resentment, criticism, and guilt
are the most damaging patterns.

Releasing resentment will dissolve even cancer.
We must release the past and forgive everyone.
We must be willing to begin to learn to love ourselves
Self-approval and self-acceptance in the now
are the keys to positive changes.

When we really love ourselves, everything in our life
works.

Even though I had hoped to climb over those difficult years
and move on in my life, there were times when my emotions
got beyond my control and I became increasingly depressed. I
reached for help from my holistic internist who prescribed
SAMe to help fight depression. For two years it helped
balance me, until without rhyme or reason, I stumbled into
an even deeper phase of gloom and felt that I needed something stronger. I wondered if the reality of my breast cancer
journey had just hit me or if it was simply the beginning of
another beginning—menopause. Looking back, I acknowledge
that it was probably a combination of those factors because
there were no apparent triggers or events for me to take a
sudden downturn. It was as if a switch had flipped inside me,
causing havoc in my brain and casting gloom on the world
around me. I simply felt lousy and could not make any
decisions about anything.

My therapist kept advising me to give myself time and
that after what I had been through it was normal to feel sad.
All I could think about was my mother and how frequently
she had been depressed when I was a child and her tendency
to inflict gloom on others. I never wanted to be a burden on
my loved ones. During the day I escaped to my writing studio

and wrote all day. At night I tossed and turned in bed, unable to fall asleep. I tried to remain upbeat and loving, but those close to me saw beyond my façade.

Being depressed became a vicious cycle. I was depressed, so I ate more and then I became more depressed because I felt fat and none of my clothes fit me. Friends who had not seen me since my surgery were surprised to notice that I had gained more than ten pounds. Most people assume that cancer victims become thinner. I became an enigma. What people did not realize was that because of the early discovery of my breast cancer, it was completely removed and I had dodged having chemotherapy and radiation. My internist reminded me that my weight gain was due to both an increased caloric intake and less exercise, both related to my low-grade depression.

Just before the two-year anniversary of my diagnosis, my sense of gloom peaked and nothing alleviated my symptoms. Even though we had scheduled weekly therapy sessions, my therapist suggested I meet with a psychiatrist who might be able to supplement our conversations with an anti-depressant. At my first meeting with the psychiatrist, I made it clear that I did not want to take any medications because of the potential side effects, such as mania, urinary retention, insomnia and lack of libido. With an air of understanding he looked at me and said, "Just be patient and we'll find the right one." He told me that it could take six weeks before the medication reached its ultimate effect.

The first medication he prescribed was a very low dose of Celexa. Even though the drug insert claimed that it would take weeks for the effects to kick-in, after the first dose I felt a cloud lift around me. Maybe it was psychosomatic, but for ten hours I sat in front of my computer writing. My focus was unparalleled. I thought about becoming the literary counter-part to Danielle Steele and the possibility of spitting out two books a year if I remained on this medication for any length of time. Its effect on me was as strong as drinking pots and pots of strong coffee.

But the drug was not a perfect match. I succumbed to its worst side effects. My heart palpitations were so powerful that I felt them even while sitting completely still. I thought my heart would eject itself from my chest cavity like a cassette from a tape player. I knew it was impossible for a heart to be ejected from the chest cavity...but mine felt as if it could. Celexa made me extremely hyper and manic. Another undesirable side effect: the loss of my libido. My sex drive had always empowered me and for the first time it dwindled to an all-time, non-existent low. So I was elated, yet non-sensual. I knew this was not the most idyllic combination. My husband swore he would rather have me happy than sensual, quite an admission for a passionate man, but I could not live with myself.

I phoned my psychiatrist and the following day his nurse phoned Wellbutrin into my local pharmacy. I had heard that this anti-depressant helped many people, including one of my favorite cousins. But, not me. Once again I was not a textbook case. Wellbutrin utterly stripped me of my creativity. The creative side of my brain (whichever side that is) became gridlocked. For the three weeks on that medication, I could not even compose a simple sentence. I sat for hours gazing blankly at my computer screen, trying to find different ways to get my thoughts down, but to no avail.

Behind our bedroom doors I wanted and needed Simon to hold me and be intimate, but because of the medication, I could not go beyond that. It was as if a barrier came down forbidding me to culminate our lovemaking. I cried in Simon's arms. He told me that everything would be okay, but the frustrations continued to burrow a hole in my psyche. The loss of libido was most frustrating because it tapped into yet another loss pertaining to my womanhood.

I felt like a failure twice over.

In general, both anti-depressants transformed my mind. The emotional channel in my brain was temporarily obliterated. I became insensitive to the feelings of others, irrational and a monster to my family. I blurted comments to Simon that I would never have ordinarily made.

Once again I phoned my psychiatrist and told him that in spite of everything I was doing, including yoga and meditation classes, the side effects were unbearable. I told him that I wanted to move onto the next chapter of my life. I wanted to be set free from the mind-altering medications that changed me into the person I never wanted to be. For me it became a case of mind over matter.

This wise psychiatrist, or shrink as he sometimes called himself, admitted that in addition to time, the best healer for me was writing. Up to this point, writing had helped me survive many of life's most difficult journeys: my grandmother's suicide, my father's death, breast cancer, and bed rest with three pregnancies. Writing forces us to scrutinize the truth. Writing is about growth and it is the writer's only means for survival. I cannot help but agree with the poet Pablo Neruda's sentiment, "writing to me is like breathing."

Dampened Creativity

Once I took an anti-depressant
but never again, thank you.

The little pill locked up my writing voice
where creating a sentence became a task

of impossible extraction. Unlike before
as lyrics were my panacea when falling
into life's darkest alleys like learning
I had breast cancer at forty-seven.

So I flushed those little yellow pills
down the toilet and found my journal

in the desk drawer, and let
my fountain pen slide across its pages.

This simple gesture cured me then
and will forever shelter me from

demons which want to continuously
slash my throat and pull away my joy.

How has breast cancer affected your personal relationships?

How would you guide others in their desire to help a woman cope with cancer, (i.e. surgery, treatments and cancer's aftermath)?

What would you say to your cancer if it just walked through the door?

Many of those who have had cancer say that cancer was not a gift, but a lesson. How do you feel about this and how has cancer affected your outlook on life?

What do you like most about being alive? What are your goals, wishes and dreams for the future?

Is there anyone in particular you would like to thank?

Epilogue – A Tale of Two Cancers

"Have no fear, Diana, have no fear."

—Alexandre Raab

In spite of efforts to accept my loss, there have still been moments when recurrent sadness surfaces. Daily events such as showers, getting dressed and making love are all reminders of my altered landscape. On low days, I feel like less of a woman.

I have grown accustomed to the intermittent muscle discomfort in my mid-back area as my body compensates for the missing muscle that was removed for the reconstruction. My fitness trainer continues to help me reinforce and strengthen that area. Bi-weekly massages help to calm muscle spasms and increase lymphatic flow, and does wonders for my psyche. I have returned to all my usual routines—working out, yoga, and cooking. Since our move from Florida to California in 2005, I have enjoyed regular hiking in the hills behind my home and daily writing. In many ways, having had breast cancer has inspired me to treasure my life and the lives of my loved ones.

A few years after my bout with breast cancer, I learned that Barbara, a friend with keen mothering sensibilities, who had faithfully brought me lunches when I was on bed rest with my first child, was dying of lung cancer. I immediately packed a suitcase and made the six-hour trip to Vancouver, where she lived. I reflected on our special moments together and thought about what I could bring her, other than myself, to provide comfort. On the taxi ride from the airport, and a few blocks from her home, we passed a flower shop with the most magical selection of orchids. I stopped the cab and bought her one. Barbara died two weeks after my visit, a few months short of what would have been her sixtieth birthday. When her husband, Jim, phoned to tell us of her passing, he said that the orchid brought so much pleasure into her life, right up until her last breath. She had insisted that its placement be in her view from the hospital bed set up in their family room. The experience forced me to further ponder my past, present and future.

The loss of my breast has also united me with other losses in my life, particularly the death of my beloved grandmother. During my recovery, I was inspired to pull from my desk drawer her yellowing typewritten journal. On those pages, my grandmother shared her story about being orphaned during World War I, and her subsequent immigrations to Vienna and the US. Once again, my father's words echoed in my head, "From all bad comes good." As part of my recovery, I enrolled in graduate school and for my final thesis used my grandmother's journal to craft a memoir, *Regina's Closet: Finding My Grandmother's Secret Journal.* Even though there was no cancer connection between my grandmother and me, many of our sensibilities were similar and we both used the power of writing as a way of healing.

After reading my grandmother's story and publishing my memoir, I decided to forge ahead with my life and not get bogged down with the genetics of my disease. I realized that it really did not matter why I got cancer or how it might have been passed on to me. The important thing was that the cancer had been removed from my body, and that I should get on with my life and continue to relish the passions that propel me forward. But even triumphs do not always have a nice neat bow wrapped around them.

In August 2006, the fifth year anniversary of my diagnosis with breast cancer, I returned to my oncologist's office in Los Angeles. He examined me and said that everything seemed fine. As he did on previous appointments, he ordered annual blood work. He sent me on my way, but three days later I received an astonishing phone call.

"Your blood protein levels are abnormally elevated and I'd like you to return for a repeat test." When I asked him what that might mean, he said that it was too early to discuss and that I should not worry.

I refrained from researching on the Internet because I really did not have enough information to go on, plus I did not want to overreact unnecessarily. Yet, I knew my husband, the scientist, did his own quiet research and the following morning, I could see worry across his face.

I returned for my blood test and the results still came back with an elevated Immunoglobulin-A (IgA). "I'm not sure what's going on," my oncologist said on the phone, not a very reassuring comment to a patient who just wanted to celebrate the anniversary of her five-year survival.

"We have to do further testing."

"Like what?"

"A bone marrow biopsy is the only definitive test."

"What might I have?"

"I want to rule out multiple myeloma."

"What's that?"

After a pregnant pause, he said, and I could almost feel him cringe as he spoke, "cancer of the plasma cells in the bone marrow."

I felt my eyes swell with tears as my mind pedaled back to five years earlier. *How could this be happening?*

"Listen, Diana. Please don't worry. Let's wait and see," he added.

Still seated at my desk, I hung up the phone and sat staring at the Edward Hopper painting on my office wall. I wanted to be the woman on the train reading. I wanted to disappear somewhere where nobody could find me. I could not bear any more bad news. "Bone marrow cancer." I said out loud, "You must be kidding!"

In slow motion I transported myself to my reading chair and ruminated about how anything could possibly be wrong with me again. I had survived breast cancer, and although I had dodged chemotherapy and radiation, I was still living with the aftermath of a mastectomy and reconstruction. For the previous five years I had been followed by my holistic internist, had eaten organically, practiced meditation, swallowed a plethora of herbs and minerals, and exercised on a regular basis. There were those who were less diligent about their physical and mental well being who showed no signs of disease. I felt doomed.

Four days after the bone marrow biopsy, my oncologist phoned to say that my diagnosis was confirmed—I officially had my second cancer in five years, and even though it was not my other breast, as I had initially feared, I now had a type of cancer that was potentially more serious. I had smoldering multiple myeloma. Unlike breast cancer, this type of cancer could not be excised from my body. It also could not be cured. I would have to live with it for the rest of my life.

When I asked if there was any connection between my history of breast cancer and multiple myeloma, he said "not to my knowledge; it has not been linked." He went on to try to comfort me by saying, "Chances are you'll die from something else." He told me to make believe that I did not have the disease. His recommendations were absolutely impossible to execute! How could I live a normal life when one day my bone marrow might get so full of bad blood cells that my bones could possibly fracture as a result?

I think he was equally shocked by my diagnosis. The typical profile of a person with multiple myeloma is a sixty-eight year old male who has been exposed to herbicides, petroleum products, heavy metals or asbestos. African-American men have the highest incidence and white women the lowest. After my diagnosis, I decided to seek out a world-renowned specialist in multiple myeloma. Dr. Keith Stewart practices at Mayo Clinic in Arizona. He trained in England, and has worked in prestigious facilities in both Canada and the United States. At the Mayo, he spends most of his time doing clinical research. His work is supported by the National Cancer Institute, Multiple Myeloma Research Foundation, Leukemia & Lymphoma Society, as well as with some pharmaceutical industries. He only follows a few select patients and so I see myself as one of the lucky ones.

Being under the joint care of my integrative medical physician and Dr. Stewart has given me the confidence I need to survive yet another cancer and dodge the chemotherapy bullet, but all I can really do is live in hope.

I have only done a sparse amount of reading about multiple myeloma because I do not want to know too much. I only want to know the basics: this is a cancer of the plasma cells in the bone marrow and the malignant plasma cells or myeloma cells accumulate in the bone marrow and cause small localized tumors that grow inside or outside the bone. The accumulation of these cells in the bone marrow can result in various problems, such as anemia, destruction of the surrounding bone, excess protein in the urine and a decrease in immune function. This is because as plasma cells increase there is less room for white blood cells to fight disease. Therefore, the person's immune system is compromised.

The incidence of multiple myeloma is about one in 100,000 Americans and approximately 15,000 cases are diagnosed each year.

I will never forget certain things people told me when I was first diagnosed with multiple myeloma. Dr. Lawrence Piro, the oncologist responsible for identifying my myeloma said: "If this condition or experience does not rivet your focus on life, then you've missed the point."

His words have resonated more and more with me over the past three years —they inspire me to live every day as if it were my last, with a sense of urgency. I realize that there are so many books I want to write and places I want to visit. I refuse to let this second diagnosis dampen my dreams.

Another comment that continues to resonate with me was made by my father-in-law, a man I have loved and admired for over thirty-five years. "Have no fear, Diana, have no fear," he told me, "that's how I survived all my life's tragedies and that's how you should get through yours." And now as this wise, strong family patriarch battles the effects of Parkinson's disease, his words become more powerful in my mind. Each and every day I try to honor his wisdom and forge ahead with my life as if I were perfectly healthy.

My holistic internist continues to take every precaution to keep me healthy. Because my immune system is somewhat compromised, I take an array of vitamins, minerals, and herbs and try to stay clear from those who are sick. I have also made a habit of regular hand-washing. Last year, before traveling to Africa with my family, I received all the typical vaccinations, plus a two-week prophylactic course of antibiotics to avoid getting any infections that could severely tax my immune system.

This year marks four years after my second cancer diagnosis and I am happy to report that, although my blood protein levels remain high, I feel better than ever. I take all the necessary precautions to remain as healthy as possible. By keeping my stress levels down, exercising, meditating, and eating well, the specialists say that it might be a long time, if ever, that I might be a candidate for treatment. In the meantime, research teams like Dr. Stewart's are working hard to develop better and more efficient treatments for multiple myeloma.

I try to remain optimistic and only focus on the disease in the days before my visit to the Mayo Clinic. Obviously, the physicians cannot make promises or predictions, especially because I am not a typical myeloma patient. I must realistically understand that things can change at any time or in the years ahead. Still, I try to live in the moment and not allow my unknown future to dominate my present. Sometimes I succumb to panic attacks, particularly when I am sad or miss my children who now all live on the East Coast. To help me through emotionally difficult moments, I speak regularly with my therapist. She continues to be supportive, keeps an eye on my elevated protein levels, and helps me deal with the present and future eventualities.

There is no doubt that having been diagnosed with two cancers in eight years has cast a new light on my life. My goal is not to let these health issues control how I live, but rather to allow them to add to it. I want to continue being productive and making my loved ones happy and proud. This is a choice that I promise to live up to.

My family has been supportive and loving during these early stages of my new disease. My husband copes by reading about the disease and gets some comfort from knowing what to expect. My children cope by channeling their energies into their work and creativity. However, I know that once in a while they have moments of fear when they question my mortality. During those times, they will quietly ask my husband how I am doing. Usually, these fears surface around the time of my oncologist appointments and/or when one of their friends' parents have passed away, or during the holidays. This truly brings the fear home to their hearts.

Although at first I thought that multiple myeloma was insurmountable, I now realize that I can continue to live my life much the same as before my diagnosis. My plan is to survive this new hurdle of surprises my body has sprung on me. My history shows that I am a fighter. To quote Nietzsche, "That which does not kill us makes us stronger."

There are a number of messages I have taken from the cancer journey, but, for me, the most important one is that the diagnosis of cancer should be considered a turning point that sets you free to fulfill or examine dreams that can no longer wait. It can be a time when you feel infinite strength and are prompted to look inside yourself not only for ways to cope, but for secrets to your own happiness. It is about understanding what you really want in life. Many times, this means reaching back into your childhood to examine what your passions were back then. Some of your secrets may lie in those years. My family and friends always encouraged my writing because they understand its healing powers. In a profound way, having cancer brought out the poet in me, which had been dormant since my youth. For this I am so thankful.

In spite of everything, I try to wake up every morning happy to be alive and with joy in my heart. I believe it is very important to surround myself with those who bring only positive and nurturing energy into my life. Being surrounded by joy brings joy and helps you move forward toward your dreams.

Naked

When my body decided to get sick again,
six sinus infections since last birthday,
I marched into the best ENT specialist,
waiting room lined with Hollywood's
finest stars begging for reasons why they
couldn't reach the octave of the day before,
impatiently flipping through old magazines,
interrupted by cell phones ringing in unison.

I got the lead role, thanks for your inquiry,
want to go to Hawaii for the weekend? Susie
died. Funeral tomorrow. Allan's away on business,
This doctor sucks. I have lunch with Ellen at noon.
Dad's in the hospital. Freckles just had pups, want one?

My name is called. I shuffle behind the nurse,
my chart clasped to her chest like the baby
she might never have had, into the shoebox-sized room
packed with instruments I didn't know,
despite three years of nursing school.

The suave, forty-something doctor
released my X-rays from their sleeve,
and mounted them onto a screen.
He looked up through his sleek wire frames,
"You're absolutely beautiful on the outside,
but a mess on the inside." I wondered if
he was making a pass or soliciting
a surgical procedure and how many times
he repeated that line, loud enough for

the pedestrians five floors down to hear
this and the other truths about my battlefields—
three C-sections, knee surgery, twice a victim
of what strikes one in eight women, and reconstructed
organs of sensuality with tattoos to hide their truths.

Now I dodge doctors as one avoids the cones
at the scene of an accident, but I can't dodge this one.
My voice is hoarse, my breathing is short.
I envy those vacuous starlets in the waiting room,
listening to their chitter-chatter on cell phones. I sit
before the surgeon who tells me one more time,
something I need to do to hang onto my life,
but I'd rather be the person before the scalpel found me.

Sauna Poetics

Waves of agony trickle
from my skin as I sit
sweaty beneath these
roasting lights which
promise to cook the
toxins from me like
a lobster gently lowered
into its boiling water.

My bones, which carry these
malignant cells, stand up
to face another day in a
life where all we wish for is
that their genetics don't
become heir to grandchildren
who've not yet been born.

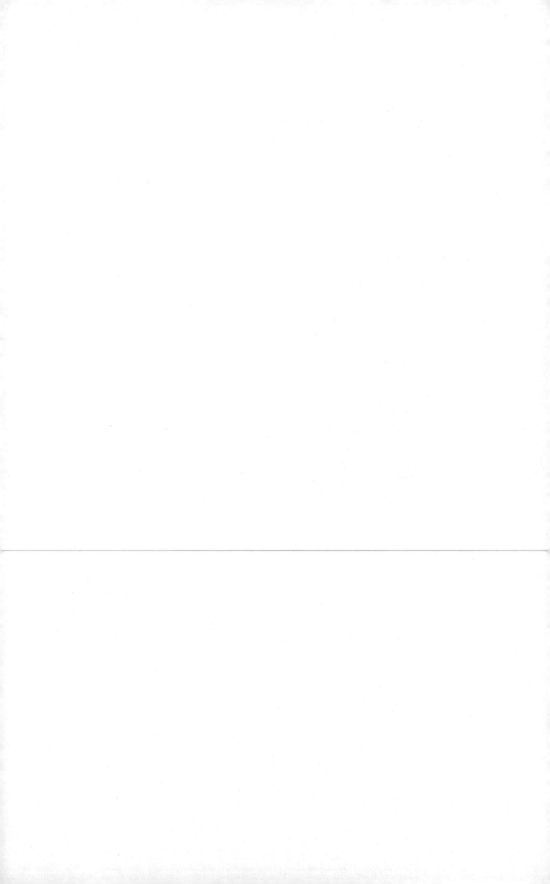

Appendix A – Writing For Wellness

There have been many books written about how to cope with the emotional aspect of illness. Most of them are the work of therapists who have studied the survivors of both acute and chronic diseases. I am not a therapist nor a counselor, but I am a nurse, educator and cancer survivor with enough experience to teach you how to use writing for healing.

Over the years, studies have shown that writing down your feelings can improve communication, enhance immune function, improve lung function, decrease stress, facilitate healing, and improve mood and general well-being.

Other benefits of keeping a notebook include:
- The notebook is a companion and best friend.
- The notebook is a place to record and remember events.
- The notebook nurtures the creative spirit.
- The notebook increases awareness.
- The notebook clears the mind.
- The notebook builds self-confidence.
- The notebook allows self-expression.
- The notebook is a safe place to vent bottled-up emotions.
- The notebook connects us with our inner voices.
- The notebook encourages reflection.
- The notebook invites imagination.
- The notebook is an emotional release.

Whether you call it a notebook, diary, journal or daybook, it is a place to heal, to document actions, reactions and observations during difficult times and turning points. Some exercises and prompts will resonate with you more than others. There is no correct way to keep a notebook. You must do what works well for you.

Some people write more easily than others. For those who need guidance, the following pages contain some meditative and inspirational quotations to help inspire you to get your words on the page. The quotations will also help you develop a positive attitude as you heal from your illness. After filling up these pages, go out and buy yourself a journal you love— one that you enjoy holding and looking at.

The Writing Process

The best way to start writing is to find a notebook or journal that resonates with you. It should lie completely flat and the pages should be easy to write on. Then also choose a pen that glides comfortably across the page. Find a place to write where you feel comfortable. Some people like starting with a centering ritual, for example lighting a candle, burning incense, having a cup of tea, exercising, showering or meditating. These practices get you in the mood for beginning your journaling practice.

When you first begin your writing routine, it is a good idea to begin with twenty minutes a day, preferably the same time every day. Many people find it easiest to write first thing in the morning when thoughts are clearer.

Always date your entries. Begin by free-writing or writing about the first thing that comes to your mind. Do not lift your pen off the page. It is okay if one thought leads to another. Go with the flow of your words. Do not edit yourself, make judgments or cross out.

If you do not know what to write, then you can start by writing over and over again, "I don't know what to write." It is amazing how your thoughts will suddenly come to you. You can also start writing about an emotional upheaval or event that is bothering you.

You should be aware of the 'flip-out rule,' devised by Dr. James W. Pennebaker in his book, *Writing to Heal.* He says this: "If you feel your writing about a particular topic is too much for you to handle, then do not write about it. If you know that you aren't ready to address a particular painful topic, write about something else. When you are ready, then tackle it. If you feel that you will flip out by writing, don't write."

Writing is one of the best ways to deal with unresolved traumas from the past. At first, you may feel as if you are back in the traumatic situation, but you should keep in mind that you are safe if you are re-experiencing the emotions. Eventually the distress will fade and might permanently disappear. In the end, this means that you have been working through the pain and not avoiding it.

Here are some ideas to write about:
- Write a letter to a loved one expressing your feelings
- Make a list of all the wonderful things about yourself
- Make a list about your biggest challenges and pick one or two to write about in depth
- Make a list of 100 reasons to be happy
- Make a list of 100 things that make you mad
- Make a list of 100 things you want to accomplish
- Write what you think about the saying, "From all bad comes good."

In addition to the prompts at the end of each chapter, it is also fun to write your feelings or insights about well-known quotes. You can choose your own favorite quotes or use some of the ones on the following pages:

"Nature's way of healing is through deep rest."

Thomas Crum

"Remember that all things pass. If worry comes—it is a passing thing."

Hazrat Inayat Khan

"Laughter is by definition healthy."

Doris Lessing

"The words that enlighten the soul are more precious than jewels."

Hazrat Inayat Khan

Write on!

It's for you.

It's for your health.

It's for your life!

Appendix B – Healing Pages

Healing begins from within and in many cases is controlled by our minds. If we can achieve a sense of calm and acceptance about our disease, then healing will ensue. Lately, there has been a great deal written about the mind-body connection and I cannot overemphasize its importance.

The first step in healing or achieving a positive mind-body connection is to maintain a sense of mindfulness. This means having a concentrated awareness of one's thoughts, activities and motivations. It also means living in the moment and realizing that thoughts are just thoughts. When you realize this then it will be easier to understand and cope with reality.

During my own breast cancer journey, I used various modalities to try to establish a sense of mindfulness about my situation. I frequently listened to new age, calming music, I mediated and journaled. All these methods helped to guide me. Before using any of these modalities, I taught myself to enter a deep state of relaxation.

RELAXATION

Entering a deep state of relaxation involves trusting yourself. You have to want to let go and believe in the benefits of bringing calm into your life. The two most common positions for relaxing are either lying down or sitting, whichever is more comfortable for you.

You will slowly feel quite relaxed. Keep in mind that the body heals when both the mind and body are relaxed. The art of relaxation does not happen immediately. You must practice it regularly.

Prone Position

This involves lying flat on your back either on the floor or on your bed. Do not use a pillow. Your legs should be extended and your feet should be about twelve inches apart. Your arms should be outstretched from your body and your palms face up. Make sure you are dressed warmly because when you are relaxed, there is a tendency to become chilled.

Next, close your eyes. Take some long and deep breaths. Each time you exhale, you should feel your body sinking into the ground or mattress. Then, starting with your feet, begin by focusing on each part of your body. With each breath allow each part of your body to relax. Once you have made it all the way from your feet up to your head, continue the rhythmic breathing. Allow your mind to go blank. Do not allow yourself to become obsessed with any images or thoughts. You might find yourself drifting off into sleep and this is fine. Do not worry if thoughts come into your mind. This is normal. Allow them to be there, but just don't pay attention to them.

Seated Position

If you prefer the seated position for relaxation, then you can sit on a cushion placed on the floor keeping your back as straight as possible. Some people prefer using meditation chairs. Rest your hands on your lap or place them face down on your thighs. It's critical to keep your back straight.

MEDITATION

Meditation has been practiced for thousand of years. There are many different types of practice. The type of meditation that has been advocated for wellness is called 'mindful meditation.' It involves being conscious about what is going on, while paying attention and not reacting to your situation or the environment. When your body is in a state of relaxation, it becomes more connected with its core. Meditation helps you learn how to accept what is going on, rather than reacting to it. It's the reaction segment that results in unnecessary stress on your body.

Some people like beginning their meditation with a centering ritual, such as lighting a white candle. After your centering ritual, begin to meditate by closing your eyes. Become aware of your position and imagine your body as an envelope and that you are inside it. Allow yourself to be inside your body. Remain in the moment. Now, start focusing on your breath. Notice which is the strongest part of your breath—the inhale or the exhale. You can figure this out by focusing on your diaphragm and how it rises and falls.

Continue to concentrate on your breath. If you feel your mind wandering to an image or thought, bring your attention back to your breath. Your breath should be the focus of your thoughts.

In the beginning you can start with a five-minute meditation session, but soon your five minutes may become 10, 15 or 20. You will find yourself looking forward to your quiet time and the sense of calm you feel afterward. You should practice meditation at least once each day, preferably at the same time. The more you can make the practice a habit, the better your results will be.

Appendix C – Glossary

185delAG – a genetic mutation carried by Ashkenazi Jews which can cause a susceptibility to breast and ovarian cancer.

acidic - any chemical compound that, when dissolved in water, gives a solution with a pH of less than 7.

alkaline - a specific type of base, which is soluble in water.

anemia – a decrease in the number of normal red blood cells.

anesthesia – the process of blocking the perception of pain and other sensations, allowing a patient to undergo surgery without the distress and pain they would otherwise experience.

aspiration - putting a hypodermic needle into tissue and drawing back on the syringe to obtain fluid or cells.

atypia - clinical term for abnormality in a cell.

attention deficit disorder (ADD) - a syndrome characterized by short attention span and hyperactivity.

biopsy - a medical test that involves the removal of tissue for the purpose of microscopic examination. The amount of tissue removed varies depending on the type of biopsy.

breast reconstruction - the creation of an artificial breast by a plastic surgeon, done either immediately after or soon after mastectomy.

calcifications - small calcium deposits in the breast tissue that may be seen by mammography.

Celexa – an antidepressant which rebalances serotonin levels to help improve moods. It's in a group of drugs called selective serotonin reuptake inhibitors (SSRI's).

cesarean - a form of childbirth in which a surgical incision is made through the mother's abdomen and uterus; typically performed when vaginal delivery could lead to medical complications.

chemotherapy - treatment of disease with certain chemicals; typically referring to cytotoxic drugs given for cancer treatment.

diagnosis - the process of identifying a medical condition or disease by its signs, symptoms, and results of diagnostic procedures. The conclusion reached through this process is called a diagnosis.

diffuse - widely spread or scattered; dispersed.

duct - a tubular bodily channel or passage, especially one for carrying a glandular secretion.

ductal – related or belonging to a duct.

ductal carcinoma in situ - the most common type of noninvasive breast cancer in women occurring within the milk ducts. "*In situ*" means the cancer cells have not grown outside their site of origin; sometimes referred to as pre-cancer.

ductal hyperplasia – a medical condition where cells in the milk ducts of the breast undergo abnormal growth.

expander method - a method of breast reconstruction whereby a hollow sac is placed behind the chest muscle and sewn closed. A little tube and valve is then attached to the sac, and over the course of three to six months, the surgeon injects increasing amounts of saline solution until the sac is completely full. When the sac reaches the desired size, it is removed.

glandular system - pertaining to the body's glands which are usually secretionary organs or structures.

hyperplasia - excessive growth of cells.

immunoglobulin-A - an antibody produced in the mucous membranes which plays an important role in mucosal immunity.

in situ - means the cancer cells have not grown outside their site of origin; sometimes referred to as pre-cancer.

intraductal - within the duct; can describe a benign or malignant process.

latissimus dorsi flap - flap of skin and muscle taken from the mid-back and used for breast reconstruction following a mastectomy.

mammary duct - a tubular channel within the breast.

mammogram - an X-ray film of the breast tissue used to diagnose tumors and cysts. They have been proven to reduce mortality from breast cancer.

mastectomy - the medical term for the surgical removal of one or both breasts, either partially or completely.

maxoplexy - uplift of the breast performed by a plastic surgeon.

multiple myeloma - cancer of the plasma cells in the bone marrow which are crucial for immune system function because they are responsible for antibody production.

myocutaneous flap - flap of skin, muscle and fat taken from one part of the body to fill in an empty space. For breast reconstruction, the most common site is the abdomen.

needle biopsy - the removal of a small amount of tissue or cellular material with a long hollow surgical needle, performed for diagnostic purposes.

nervous system - bodily system that coordinates muscle activity, monitors the organs, constructs and also stops input from the senses and initiates actions. All parts of the nervous system are made of nervous tissues.

oncologist - a physician who studies cancer.

pH - used to express the acidity or alkalinity of a solution on a scale of 0 to 14, where less than 7 represents acidity, 7 neutrality, and more than 7 alkalinity.

post-operative - after an operation.

prognosis - expected or probable outcome.

psychotropic - a chemical substance that acts primarily upon the central nervous system altering brain function, resulting in temporary changes in perception, mood, consciousness and behavior.

radiation - a process of emission of energy in the form of waves or particles; used to eradicate cancer.

radiology - the medical specialty directing medical imaging technologies to diagnose and sometimes treat diseases.

reconstructive surgery - surgery to reconstruct damaged or malformed tissues or organs.

saline - a sterile solution of sodium chloride; sometimes given intravenously as a medium to dilute medications.

SAMe – a synthetic form of a compound found in the body used to treat depression by increasing the availability of serotonin and dopamine.

urologist - a physician who treats conditions and diseases of the urinary tracts of both males and females.

Wellbutrin - an antidepressant medication sometimes used to help stop smoking.

Appendix D – Cancer Support Organizations

African American Breast Cancer Alliance
(612) 825-3675
www.aabcainc.org

American Breast Cancer Foundation
(877) 539-2543
www.abcf.org

American Cancer Society
(800) ACS-2345
www.cancer.org

American Society of Clinical Oncology
(571) 483-1300
www.asco.org

American Society of Plastic Surgeons
www.plasticsurgery.org

BreastCancer.org
www.breastcancer.org

The Breast Cancer Fund
(415) 346-8223
www.breastcancerfund.org

Breast Cancer Network of Strength
(800) 221-2141
www.networkofstrength.org

California Breast Cancer Organizations
(530) 304-2746
www.cabco-org.us

Cancer Network
www.cancernetwork.com

Cancer Research Institute
(800) 99-CANCER
www.cancerresearch.org

Cancer Support Community
(888) 793-WELL
www.thewellnesscommunity.org

Chemocare
www.chemocare.com

The Chemotherapy Foundation
(212) 213-9292
www.chemotherapyfoundation.org

Corporate Angel Network, Inc.
(914) 328-1313
www.corpangelnetwork.org

International Cancer Alliance
(301) 656-3461
www.icare.org

Johns Hopkins Avon Foundation Breast Cancer Center
(443) 287-**2778**
www.hopkinsbreastcenter.org

Kids Konnected
(800) 899-2866
www.kidskonnected.org

Lance Armstrong Foundation
(877) 236-8820
www.livestrong.com

Leukemia and Lymphoma Society
(800) 955-4572
www.leukemia-lymphoma.org

Living Beyond Breast Cancer
(888) 753-5222
www.lbbc.org

The Mautner Project for Lesbians with Cancer
(202) 332-5536
www.mautnerproject.org

Mothers Supporting Daughters with Breast Cancer
(410) 778-1982
www.mothersdaughters.org

Multiple Myeloma Research Foundation
(203) 229-0464
www.themmrf.org

Myriad Genetics & Laboratories
(801) 584-3600
www.myriad.com

National Asian Women's Health Organization
www.nawho.org

National Breast Cancer Coalition
(202) 296-7477
www.stopbreastcancer.org

National Cancer Coalition
www.nationalcancercoalition.org

National Cancer Institute
(800) 4-CANCER
www.cancer.gov

National Center for Complementary and Alternative Medicine
(888) 644-6226
www.nccam.nih.gov

National Cervical Cancer Coalition
(800) 685-5531
www.nccc-online.org

National Coalition for Cancer Survivorship
(888) 650-9127
www.canceradvocacy.org

National Comprehensive Cancer Network
www.nccn.org

National Lymphedema Network
(800) 541-3259
www.lymphnet.org

National Marrow Donor Program
www.marrow.org

National Women's Health Network
(202) 682-2640
www.nwhn.org

Native American Cancer Research
(800) 537-8295
www.natamcancer.org

Office of Minority Health Resource Center
(800) 444-6472
www.minorityhealth.hhs.gov

OncoChat
www.oncochat.org

Oncology Nursing Society
(866) 257-4667

www.ons.org

Patient Advocate Foundation
(800) 532-5274

www.patientadvocate.org

R.A. Bloch Cancer Foundation
(800) 433-0464

www.blochcancer.org

Sisters Network, Inc.
(866) 781-1808

www.sistersnetworkinc.org

Dr. Susan Love Research Foundation
(866) 569-0388

www.dslrf.org

Susan G. Komen Breast Cancer Foundation
(877) 465-6636

www.komen.org

Vital Options TeleSupport Cancer Network
(818) 508-5657

www.vitaloptions.org

Young Survival Coalition
(877) YSC-1011

www.youngsurvival.org

About the Author

Diana M. Raab, MFA, RN is a memoirist and poet and author of six books. She teaches in the UCLA Extension Writers' Program and at various conferences around the country. She is a member of the American Medical Writers' Association (AMWA), the Author's Guild and Poets & Writers. Her award-winning writing has appeared in numerous national publications and anthologies.

Diana was born in Brooklyn and raised in Queens, New York. She earned her BSc in Health Administration with a minor in Journalism from Cortland State University in 1997. She pursued a nursing degree from Vanier College and was a Director of Nursing in Montreal, Canada. She then received a positive pregnancy test followed by her doctor's prescription for bed rest. As a result, she resigned from her administrative position and became a freelance medical writer, which resulted in over 300 published articles to her credit. While on bed rest, she chronicled her experience, which evolved into a self-help book called, *Getting Pregnant and Staying Pregnant: Overcoming Infertility and High-Risk Pregnancy* which has been in print since 1988 and has been translated into French and Spanish. In 1992, it won the Benjamin Franklin Book Award for Best Health and Wellness Book.

In 2009, Diana updated this book in collaboration with Errol Norwitz, M.D., Professor, Yale University School of Medicine and Co-Director, Division of Maternal-Fetal Medicine, Yale New Haven Hospital and was published by

Hunter House under the new title, *Your High Risk Pregnancy: A Practical and Supportive Guide.*

After recovering from breast cancer in 2003, Diana returned to school for her Masters in Writing at Spalding University's Low-Residency Program. Her thesis was the basis of her memoir, *Regina's Closet: Finding My Grandmother's Secret Journal* (Beaufort Books, 2007) which received numerous high honors, including the 2009 Mom's Choice Award for Best Adult Nonfiction and the 2008 National Indie Award for Best Memoir. This memoir is based on the story of Diana discovering her grandmother's secret journal more than three decades after she took her life in Diana's childhood home. Regine, Diana's glamorous and spirited grandmother, loved and cared for Diana until she was ten. The book discusses coming to grips with her grandmother's suicide and her family's history of depression.

During her MFA program Diana also began a second memoir, which focused on her breast cancer journey, and which ultimately resulted in this book, *Healing With Words: A Writer's Cancer Journey.* This book was written with the hope of encouraging women to journal through their own cancer saga. Since writing has always helped her navigate through tumultuous times in her life, Diana advocates journaling as a way of healing.

Diana has three books of poetry, *My Muse Undresses Me* (2007), *Dear Anaïs: My Life in Poems for You* (2008) and *The Guilt Gene* (2009). She's editor of the anthology, *Writers and Their Notebooks* (2010) with a foreword by Phillip Lopate.

Diana's passions also include reading, yoga, hiking and traveling. Diana is married to Simon Raab and they live with their Maltese dog, Spunky, in Southern California. They have three grown children, Rachel, Regine and Joshua, with whom they are very close.

Diana's website is http://www.dianaraab.com.

Bibliography

Bodai, Ernie, M.D. and Judi Fertig Panneton. *The Breast Cancer Book of Strength and Courage: Inspiring Stories to See You Through.* New York, NY: Crown Publishing Group. 2002.

Clark, Annabel, Lynn Redgrave and Baron Lerner. *Journal: A Mother and Daughter's Recovery from Breast Cancer.* New York, NY: Powerhouse Books. 2004.

Davis, Sherry, L. *Thriving After Breast Cancer: Essential Healing Exercises for Body and Mind.* New York, NY: Broadway Books. 2002.

Drescher, Fran. *Cancer Schmancer.* New York, NY: Warner Books. 2003.

Fead, Beverlye Hyman. *I Can Do This: Living with a cancer tracing a year of hope.* Santa Barbara, CA: Santa Barbara Cancer Center. 2004.

Fisher, Ann Kempner. *B.O.O.B.S.: A Bunch of Outrageous Breast Cancer Survivors Tell Their Stories of Courage, Hope and Healing.* Nashville, TN: Cumberland Publishing Co. 2004.

Hawkins, Beth. *I'm Too Young to Have Breast Cancer!* Washington: Regnery Publishing Inc. 2004.

Hay, Louise L. *You Can Heal Your Life.* Carlsbad: CA: Hay House. 1984.

Hirshaut, Yashar and Peter Pressman. *Breast Cancer: The Complete Guide.* New York, NY: Bantam Books. 2004.

Kaye, Ronnie. *Spinning Straw Into Gold.* New York, NY: Simon and Shuster. 2002.

Lee, John R., David Zava and Virginia Hopkins. *What Your Doctor May Not Tell You About Breast Cancer.* New York, NY: Warner Books. 2002.

Link, John R., Cynthia Forsthoff and James Waisman. *The Breast Cancer Survival Manual.* New York, NY: Henry Holt & Co. 2003.

Link, John, M.D. *Take Charge of Your Breast Cancer.* New York, NY: Henry Holt & Co. 2002.

Lorde, Audre. *The Cancer Journals.* San Francisco, CA: Aunt Lute Books. 1980.

Love, Susan M. *Dr. Susan Love's Breast Book* 3rd edition. Cambridge, MA: Perseus Publishing. 2000.

McFadden, Bernice L. *Camilla's Roses.* New York, NY: Dutton Adult. 2004.

Mack, Stan. *Janet and Me: An Illustrated Story of Love and Loss.* New York, NY: Simon and Shuster. 2004.

Murray, Lorraine. *Why Me? Why Now?: Finding Hope When You Have Breast Cancer.* Notre Dame, IN: Ave Maria Press. 2003.

Pennebaker, James. W. *Writing To Heal: A Guided Journal for Recovering From Trauma & Emotional Upheaval.* Oakland, CA: New Harbinger Publications, Inc. 2004.

Raz, Hilda, ed. *Living On the Margins.* New York, NY: Persea Books. 1999.

Rollin, Betty. *Last Wish.* New York, NY: Public Affairs. 1998.

Steligo, Kathy. *The Breast Reconstruction Guidebook: Issues and Answers from Research to Recovery.* San Carlos, CA: Carlo Press. 2005.

Wadler, Joyce. *My Breast.* New York, NY: Pocket Books 1997.

Williams, Terri Tempest. *Refuge: An Unnatural History of Family and Place.* New York, NY: Vintage Books 1992.

3 1125 00695 9454

LaVergne, TN USA
02 September 2010
195445LV00001B/65/P

9 781615 990108